Manual of H ✔ KT-130-475
Management

Manual of Heart Failure Management

Edited by

John D. Bisognano, Marc L. Baker, and Mary Beth Earley

Department of Medicine, Cardiology Division,
University of Rochester, Rochester, NY, USA

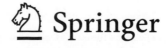 Springer

Editors
John D. Bisognano, MD, PhD
Department of Medicine
Cardiology Division
University of Rochester
Rochester, NY
USA

Marc L. Baker, MD, PhD
Department of Medicine
Cardiology Division
University of Rochester
Rochester, NY
USA

Mary Beth Earley, CCRN, MS, NP
Department of Medicine
Cardiology Division
University of Rochester
Rochester, NY
USA

ISBN 978-1-84882-184-2   e-ISBN 978-1-84882-185-9
DOI: 10.1007/978-1-84882-185-9
Springer Dordrecht Heidelberg London New York

British Library Cataloguing in Publication Data
A catalogue record for this book is available from the British Library

Library of Congress Control Number: PCN applied for

Printed on acid-free paper

Springer is part of Springer Science+Business Media (www.springer.com)

Preface

Heart failure (HF) is a chronic progressive disease with less than 50% of patients living five years after their initial diagnosis and less than 25% are alive at 10 years. Our current system of HF care, which is characterized by a cycle of acute hospitalizations and acute episodic outpatient care by a primary or emergency room provider, has not led to great improvement in patient quality of life or prognosis. Our Healthcare System will triage and diagnose acute illness and get professional treatment as soon as possible. The role of the patients is largely passive, the role of the caregivers is microscopically focused, and the time course of the hospital experience is much shorter than the insidious development of HF. When patients with decompensated HF were followed after discharge from an emergency department community Hospital, 61% returned to the emergency department or were admitted to the hospital within 3 months and had a median time to failure of 30 days. In a recent population-based cohorts study, one third of all patients admitted to the emergency department returned for at least one more emergency room visit. Two thirds of all patients were admitted to the hospital and 20% died within the first year. Self-management skills are critical to progression of care in any chronic disease state, and the patient has little incentive to develop self-management skills in the Emergency Room. Assessing prognosis in HF is the subject of much research, and compared with other chronic disease states this has proven very difficult, particularly in HF with preserved left ventricular systolic function. What is certain is that HF is a chronic progressive disease with less than 50% of patients living five years after their initial diagnosis and less than 25% are alive at 10 years. Furthermore, the mortality of HF is not understood by the general public. Using a

1991 Scottish database, 16,224 men had an initial hospitalization for HF (n = 3,241), myocardial infarction (n = 6,932) or cancer of the lung, large bowel, prostate, or bladder (n = 6,051). Similarly, 14,842 women were admitted for HF (n = 3,606), myocardial infarction (n = 4,916), or cancer of the breast, lung, large bowel, or ovary (n = 6,320). With the exception of lung cancer, HF was associated with the poorest 5-year survival rate (approximately 25% for both sexes). On an adjusted basis, HF was associated with worse long-term survival than bowel cancer in men and breast cancer in women. HF is as "malignant" as many common types of cancer and is associated with a comparable number of expected life-years lost. It is critical to obtain patient understanding of their disease progression, utilizing the known stages of NYHA Functional Class and AHA/ACC Stages to allow accurate communication between all the different levels of caregivers. Furthermore, the education of patients as well as the emergency department and primary care physicians remains a formidable barrier to HF care.

For patients receiving optimal treatment, NYHA class determined during periods of clinical stability correlates with prognosis. Mortality is 5–10% per year in patients with class I symptoms, and increases to 40–50% per year for those with class IV symptoms. Functional status is also a strong predictor, tending to decline over the 3 months prior to death. However, NYHA Class as determined by physicians, not direct patient reported questionnaires is what correlates with prognosis. Physician input may be needed for prognosis for many reasons. Patients with EF >30% and other risk factors may have higher mortality and a higher risk of sudden death than some patients with EF ≤30%. Various other models exist for HF prognosis, some of which have been compared and validated with independent predictors of mortality. The ADHERE database revealed the importance of renal function in determining in hospital prognosis. However, independent predictors of mortality often have no meaning to treatment applications of HF, and therefore become meaningless to the caregiver. A model that predicts prognosis based on treatments does not yet exist for acute decompensated HF, but would be of tremendous use.

Our system also has trouble with the complex underlying science of HF, as well as the new technologies available. The ultimate treatment is a cardiac transplant, but the limited number of hearts available and comorbid conditions are limiting factors. Other options are not available to the general populations as of yet. The majority of treatment may actually be prevention. In the GRACE study, improvements in the management of patients with ACS were associated with significant reductions in the rates of new HF and mortality and in rates of stroke and mycoardial infarction at 6 months. In addition, prevention is only a portion of the population treatment plan. Therefore, treatment for the remaining 4.99 million clinic patients must ensue, and can be accomplished in a specialized HF Clinic.

Finally, even in a multidiscipline approach, HF often demands care beyond that of a clinical setting, and outside help is required. The purpose of this book is to unite individual foci of HF treatment and specialization into a global perception to present correctly the tremendous obstacles facing our HF patients. Each facet of HF treatment operates independently as part of another program, without realizing their importance for the "heart failure nation." Like terminal cancer, there is no cure for HF. Unlike terminal cancer, public perception of terminal HF is limited. "At least I don't have cancer," is a familiar quotation amongst HF patients. Most patients do not realize they are more likely to die from cardiovascular problems *with* their cancer. There will certainly be more patients with HF in the future. Understanding the next step of treatment beyond your own caretaker abilities is critical for patient care and education, for changing public perception, and for translating research opportunities into treatment protocols for the future.

Marc L. Baker
Rochester, NY

Contents

Contributors

Mehmet Aktaş, MD
Department of Medicine, Cardiology Division,
Electrophysiology Laboratory, University of
Rochester Medical Center, Rochester, NY, USA

Jeffrey D. Alexis, MD
Department of Medicine, Cardiology Divison,
Heart Failure and Transplantation Program,
University of Rochester School of Medicine
and Dentistry, Rochester, NY, USA

Marc L. Baker, MD, PhD
Department of Medicine, Cardiology Division,
University of Rochester, Rochester, NY, USA

Bethany Barney, RD
Heart Failure and Transplantation Program,
Strong Memorial Hospital, Rochester, NY, USA

G. Ronald Beck, MS
Ambulatory Nursing, University of Rochester
Medical Center, Rochester, NY, USA

John D. Bisognano, MD, PhD
Department of Medicine, Cardiology Division University
of Rochester Medical Center, Rochester, NY, USA

Burns C. Blaxall, PhD
Department of Medicine, Aab Cardiovascular
Research Institute, Rochester, NY, USA

Robert Block, MD, MPH
Department of Community and Preventive
Medicine and Strong Preventive Cardiology Clinic,
University of Rochester School of Medicine and
Dentistry, Rochester, NY, USA

Leway Chen, MD, MPH
Department of Medicine, Cardiology Division,
University of Rochester, Rochester, NY, USA

Joseph M. Delehanty, MD
Department of Medicine, Cardiology Division,
University of Rochester Medical Center, Rochester,
NY, USA

Mary Beth Earley, CCRN, MS, NP
Cardiology Division, University of Rochester
Medical Center, Rochester, NY, USA

Jennifer Falvey, PharmD, BCPS
Department of Pharmacy, University of Rochester
Medical Center, Rochester, NY, USA

Michael W. Fong, MD
Department of Medicine, Cardiology Division,
Heart Failure and Transplantation Program,
School of Medicine and Dentistry University
of Rochester, Rochester, NY, USA

James Gallagher, MD
Department of Medicine, Cardiology Division,
University of Rochester, Rochester, NY, USA

James J. Gangemi, MD
Department of Surgery, University of Rochester
Medical Center, Rochester, NY, USA

William Hallinan, RN, MBA, EMT-P
Artificial Heart Program, University of Rochester
Medical Center, Rochester, NY, USA

Jean Heuther, RN, MSN, CCTC
Strong Heart and Vascular Center, University of
Rochester Medical Center, Rochester, NY, USA

George L. Hicks Jr., MD
Department of Surgery, University of Rochester School
of Medicine and Dentistry, Rochester, NY, USA

Ryan J. Hoefen, MD, PhD
Department of Medicine, Cardiology Division,
University of Rochester, Rochester, NY, USA

Jaekyoung Hong, MD
Department of Medicine, Cardiology Division,
University of Rochester Medical Center,
Rochester, NY, USA

Matthew R. Jonovich, MD
Department of Medicine, University of Rochester
Medical Center, Rochester, NY, USA

Heidi Kipp, RN, MSN, ACNP-BE
Heart Failure and Transplantation Program,
Strong Memorial Hospital, Rochester, NY, USA

Laurie Kopin, MS, ANP
Preventive Cardiology, University of Rochester,
Rochester, NY, USA

Anna E. Lambert, MS
Strong Heart and Vascular Center, University of
Rochester Medical Center, Rochester, NY, USA

Vicki A. Malzewski, MS
Cardiology Division, University of Rochester Medical
Center, Rochester, NY, USA

Howard T. Massey, MD
Department of Surgery, University of Rochester
Medical Center, Rochester, NY, USA

Lisa J. Musshafen, RN, MSN
School of Nursing, University of Rochester
Medical Center, Rochester, NY, USA

Mark W. Nickels, MD
Psychiatry, University of Rochester Medical
Center, Rochester, NY, USA

Lisa Norsen, ACNP, PhD
School of Nursing, University of Rochester
Medical Center, Rochester, NY, USA

Aaron M. Olden, MD
Department of Medicine, University of Rochester
Medical Center, Rochester, NY, USA

Grzegorz Pietrasik, MD, MPH
Departments of Medicine Cardiology Division,
University of Rochester, Rochester, NY, USA

Timothy E. Quill, MD
Department of Medicine, University of Rochester
Medical Center, Rochester, NY, USA

Jill R. Quinn, PhD, RN, CS-ANP, FAHA, FNAP
School of Nursing, University of Rochester,
Rochester, NY, USA

Spencer Rosero, MD
Department of Medicine, Cardiology Division,
Electrophysiology Laboratory, University of
Rochester, Rochester, NY, USA

Dana L. Shannon, RN, MSN, ANP
Artificial Heart Program, University of Rochester
Medical Center, Rochester, NY, USA

Saadia Sherazi, MD
Community and Preventive Medicine, University
of Rochester Medical Center, Rochester, NY, USA

Eugene Storozynsky, MD, PhD
Department of Medicine, Cardiology Division,
Heart Failure and Transplantation Program
University of Rochester, Rochester, NY, USA

J. Chad Teeters, MD
Department of Medicine, Cardiology Division,
University of Rochester, Rochester, NY, USA

Gladys Velarde, MD
Department of Medicine, Cardiology Division,
The Women's Heart Program, University of
Rochester Medical Center, Rochester, NY, USA

Chapter 1
Management of Hypertension in Heart Failure

Matthew R. Jonovich and John D. Bisognano

INTRODUCTION

Epidemiology of Hypertension and Cardiovascular Disease

Hypertension is the most common chronic medical disorder in the United States. According to JNC 7 criteria, more than 65 million Americans have hypertension and an additional 25% of the population has prehypertension.[1] Despite its vast prevalence, hypertension remains highly under recognized with a full 30% of patients unaware that they have the condition.

In developed societies, blood pressure increases with age. Diastolic BP plateaus in the fifth decade and may decline thereafter but systolic BP continues to rise steadily through the seventh decade. The Framingham Heart Study estimated the 20-year risk of developing hypertension as >90% for normotensive men and women of middle age (55–65 years of age).[2] Among Americans over age 65, more than half have isolated systolic or combined systolic-diastolic hypertension.

Hypertension Morbidity and Mortality

Hypertension is a major risk factor for stroke,[3] coronary artery disease (CAD),[4] myocardial infarction,[1] congestive heart failure,[5] dementia,[6] and chronic kidney disease with clear evidence of increased risk with increasing blood pressure.[7] The relationship between blood pressure and risk of cardiovascular disease (CVD)

J.D. Bisognano et al. (eds.), *Manual of Heart Failure Management*,
DOI: 10.1007/978-1-84882-185-9_1, © Springer-Verlag London Limited 2009

is strong, continuous, and independent of other risk factors. For individuals of age 40–70 years, each increment of 20 mmHg in systolic blood pressure (SBP) or 10 mmHg in diastolic blood pressure (DBP) doubles the risk of a fatal coronary event across the entire BP range from 115/75 to 185/115 mmHg.[8]

Hypertension contributes to the pathogenesis of systolic and diastolic HF through multiple mechanisms. Hypertension increases afterload and over time leads to the development of left ventricular hypertrophy, ventricular chamber remodeling, and eventually diastolic and systolic dysfunction.[9] In addition, hypertension is a major risk factor for CAD and subsequent ischemic heart failure. Not surprisingly, hypertension is especially prevalent among patients with heart failure. The Framingham Heart Study cited hypertension as the most frequent comorbidity among patients with heart failure.[2] A significant degree of the morbidity and mortality from hypertensive disease is attributed to resultant heart failure.

Benefits of Treatment
The treatment of hypertension is highly effective in reducing cardiovascular morbidity and mortality, particularly among patients with heart failure. Randomized trials prove lowering blood pressure with antihypertensive therapy produces rapid, substantial reduction in myocardial infarction averaging 20–25% and heart failure averaging more than 50%.[10] Physicians should aggressively treat hypertension in patents with heart failure to reverse hemodynamic abnormalities, relieve symptoms, decrease disease progression, and improve patient survival.

CLASSIFICATION, DIAGNOSIS, AND EVALUATION OF HYPERTENSION
Requisite to the effective management of hypertension is the appropriate classification, timely diagnosis, and thorough evaluation of the condition.

Classification of Hypertension
The seventh report of the Joint National Committee on Prevention, Detection, Evaluation, and Treatment of High Blood Pressure defines normal blood pressure as <120/<80 mmHg. Individuals with a systolic blood pressure of 120–139 mmHg or diastolic blood pressure of 80–89 mmHg are classified as prehypertensive and are at an increased risk of progression to frank hypertension. JNC 7 defines Stage I Hypertension as a SBP 140–159 mmHg or a DBP 90–99 mmHg and Stage II Hypertension as SBP> 160 mmHg or DBP> 100 mmHg in adults ages 18 and older.[1]

Diagnosis of Hypertension
The diagnosis of hypertension is established when an elevated blood pressure is measured at two separate patient visits with at least two blood pressure measurements per visit. Blood pressure should be measured by a calibrated sphygmomanometer with an appropriate-sized cuff whose bladder encircles at least 80% of the arm. The patient must be seated quietly in a chair with both feet on the floor for 5 min and arm supported at heart level.[1] Accurate, reproducible blood pressure measurement is essential to correctly classify blood pressure and gauge response to treatment. Ambulatory blood pressure monitoring may be utilized to evaluate patients with "whitecoat hypertension," establish a patient's average BP or to assess drug resistance, hypotensive symptoms, episodic hypertension, or autonomic dysfunction.[1]

Evaluation of the Patient with Hypertension
The evaluation of a patient with hypertension must include three essential elements:

1. Lifestyle assessment to identify cardiovascular risk factors and concomitant conditions (Table 1.1)
2. Past medical history for identifiable causes of high blood pressure
3. Assessment for target end organ damage or presence of CVD

The clinician should elicit a detailed past medical history to reveal cardiovascular risk factors and screen for potential causes of hypertension. Physical examination includes measurement of BP in both arms, examination of the optic fundi, calculation of BMI, auscultation for carotid, abdominal and femoral bruits; palpation of the thyroid gland, cardiac exam, pulmonary exam, abdomen exam for enlarged kidneys, masses, or abnormal aortic pulsation; palpation of lower extremities for edema and pulses, and neurological assessment. Laboratory testing includes an electrocardiogram, urinalysis, blood glucose, hematocrit, serum potassium and calcium, estimated glomerular filtration rate, and a fasting lipid profile.

Secondary Causes of Hypertension
Approximately 5–10% of hypertension cases result from an underlying, identifiable, often correctable cause.[11] The presence of refractory elevated blood pressure, onset of hypertension before age 20, evidence of significant end organ damage, or lack of family history of hypertension require investigation of secondary causes of hypertension (Table 1.2).

TABLE 1.1. Evaluation of the patient with hypertension

Major cardiovascular disease risk factors	Target organ damage
Hypertension	Heart
Cigarette smoking	Left ventricular hypertrophy (LVH)
Obesity (BMI>30 kg/m^2)	Angina or prior myocardial infarction (MI)
Physical inactivity	Prior coronary revascularization
Dyslipidemia	Heart failure (HF)
Diabetes mellitus	Brain
Microalbuminuria or estimated GFR< 60 mL/min	Stroke or transient ischemic attack (TIA)
Age (>55 for men, >65 for women)	Chronic kidney disease
Family history of premature CVD (men< age 55 or women < age 65)	Peripheral arterial disease
	Retinopathy

Adapted from JNC 7 Express. The Seventh Report of the Joint National Committee on Prevention, Detection, Evaluation and Treatment of High Blood Pressure. May 2003. NIH Publication No. 03-5233. http:www.nhlbi.nih.gov/guidelines/hypertension/jncintro.htm.

TABLE 1.2. Secondary causes of hypertension

Condition	Clinical signs/ symptoms	Diagnostic evaluation
Acromegaly	Headaches, fatigue, visual problems, enlargement of hands, feet, tongue	Growth hormone level
Aldosteronism	Hypernatremia, hypokalemia	Ratio: plasma aldosterone to plasma renin activity, CT of adrenal glands
Coarctation of aorta	Decreased or delayed femoral pulses, abnormal chest xray	Doppler or CT imaging of aorta
Cushing's syndrome	Weight gain, fatigue, weakness, hirsutism, amenorrhea, moon facies, dorsal hump, purple striae, truncal obesity, hypokalemia	Dexamethasone-suppression test

(continued)

TABLE 1.2. (continued)

Condition	Clinical signs/ symptoms	Diagnostic evaluation
Diet effect	High salt intake Excessive alcohol intake	Trial of dietary modification
Erythropoietin side effect	Erythropoietin use in CKD Polycythemia in COPD	Trial off drug (if possible)
Hyperpara- thyroidism	Kidney stones, oste- oporosis, depression, lethargy, muscle weakness	Serum calcium
		Parathyroid hormone levels
Hyperthyroidism	Heat intolerance, weight loss, pal- pitations, systolic hypertension, exoph- thalmos tremor, tachycardia	TSH level
Medication effect	Refractory/new hypertension	Trial off drug (if possible)
		Cyclosporine(Sandimmune), tacrolimus (Prograf), corticosteroids Ibuprofen (Motrin), naproxen (Naprosyn), piroxicam (Feldene) Celecoxib (Celebrex), rofecoxib (Vioxx), valdecoxib (Bextra), Estrogen OPC's (30–35 mcg) Sibutramine (Meridia), phentermine (Adipex), ma huang (ephe- dra) Nicotine, ampheta- mines, Fludrocortisone (Florinef), Bromocriptine (Parlodel), Phenelzine (Nardil),Testosterone Pseudoephedrine
Obstructive sleep apnea	Snoring, daytime som- nolence, obesity	Sleep study
Pheochro- mocytoma	Paroxysmal hypertension, headaches, diaphore- sis, palpitations, tachycardia	Urinary catecholamine metabolites (vanillylman- delic acid, metanephrines, normetanephrines) Plasma free metanephrines

(continued)

TABLE 1.2. (continued)

Condition	Clinical signs/ symptoms	Diagnostic evaluation
Renal parenchymal disease	Renal insufficiency, atherosclerotic cardiovascular disease, edema, elevated blood urea nitrogen and creatinine levels, proteinuria	Creatinine clearance
Renovascular disease	Systolic/diastolic abdominal bruit	Renal ultrasound Magnetic resonance angiography, captopril (Capoten)-augmented radioisotopic renography, renal arteriography

TREATMENT OF HYPERTENSION IN HEART FAILURE

Treatment Goals

The risk of CVD in patients with hypertension is vastly reduced by effective antihypertensive therapy. Clinical studies show ischemic heart disease and heart failure can be prevented or reversed when aggressive targets for blood pressure are achieved.[1] For the primary prevention of CVD the consensus treatment goal for BP is <140/90 mmHg. In individuals with high risk for CVD from diabetes mellitus, chronic kidney disease, or a 10-year Framingham risk score of ≥10% a goal BP< 130/80 mmHg is advised.[1,4] Recent guidelines from the AHA include individuals with demonstrated CAD or CAD risk equivalents (carotid artery disease, peripheral arterial disease, or abdominal aortic aneurysm) among those with a target BP of <130/80 mmHg.[4]

The optimal target blood pressure for patients with heart failure has not been established. It is known that hypertension imposes an increased hemodynamic load on the failing ventricle and that small changes in afterload can produce large changes in stroke volume and cardiac output. It can be argued that very low SBP values (<120 mmHg) may be beneficial in heart failure to reduce myocardial workload and improve cardiac function. By this logic, even normotensive heart failure patients benefit from treatment to further lower systemic vascular resistance. There remains concern however, that excessive BP lowering may reduce DBP to the point it impairs coronary perfusion occurring in diastole. It is known that the coronary circulation is capable of autoregulation by vasodilation to maintain constant coronary blood flow as diastolic pressure falls. This ability of the coronary vessels to dilate in response to a falling perfusion pressure is finite. It may be reasoned that at the point of maximal vasodilation a further fall in coronary perfusion pressure would result in decreased coronary blood flow and possible ischemia. To date, this autoregulatory threshold has not been validated in humans with healthy or diseased coronary arteries and no consensus exists regarding the minimum safe level of DBP. Currently the AHA recommends a BP goal of <120/<80 for patients with heart failure but cautions against inducing falls of DBP below 60 mmHg in patients with diabetes mellitus or age greater than 60 years.[4] To achieve this aggressive blood pressure goal, a successful treatment plan must combine elements of lifestyle and pharmacologic therapy.

Lifestyle Therapy
Lifestyle modifications have been shown to reduce blood pressure, enhance antihypertensive drug efficacy, and decrease cardiovascular risk. Lifestyle modifications proven to lower BP include weight reduction in individuals who are overweight or obese,[12,13] adoption of the dietary approaches to stop hypertension (DASH) diet which is rich in potassium and calcium,[14] reduction of dietary sodium to <6 g NaCl daily,[14] and regular aerobic physical activity (at least 30 min per day most days).[15] Exercise training has been shown to reduce recurrent cardiac events in patients with LV dysfunction from ischemic heart disease and is recommended but should be done under close medical supervision.[16]

Pharmacotherapy for Hypertension
The optimal choice of antihypertensive agents remains controversial despite meta-analyses that demonstrate the amount of BP reduction is more important than choice of drug class for the primary prevention of the complications of hypertension.[17] Excellent clinical outcomes data proves lowering blood pressure with thiazide diuretics, angiotensin converting enzyme inhibitors (ACE-I), angiotensin receptor blockers (ARBs), beta blockers (BBs), and calcium channel blockers (CCBs) all reduce complications of hypertension.[3,10,18,19] Since most patients require two or more antihypertensive medications to achieve goal BP the choice of the initial agent is less important in primary prevention of CVD.[1]

In patients with heart failure not all drug classes have been proven to confer the same benefit. ACE inhibitors, ARBs, beta blockers, and aldosterone antagonists have favorable effects on survival that are independent of their effects on blood pressure. Specific medication choices must be tailored to the type of heart failure present in the patient. Systolic heart failure is a state of impaired cardiac contractility diagnosed by decreased left ventricular ejection fraction. The goals of antihypertensive therapy in systolic dysfunction are to diminish congestive symptoms by reducing preload and to improve cardiac contractility by reducing afterload. Diuretics, ACE inhibitors, beta blockers, and aldosterone agonists all improve survival in systolic heart failure. Diastolic heart failure results from poor diastolic filling and decreased forward output due to increased ventricular stiffness with preserved LVEF. Optimal antihypertensive therapy in diastolic dysfunction is uncertain, but beta blockers, ACE inhibitors, and ARBs may be beneficial.

When formulating a successful treatment plan the clinician must consider the type of heart failure present, weigh the benefits of each class of medication based on best evidence available, and consider the use of generic medications to reduce prescription costs (Table 1.3).

Thiazide Diuretics

Thiazide diuretics are highly effective in reducing blood pressure and preventing ischemic heart failure in patients with hypertension.[18] Thiazide type diuretics are recommended for patients with mild HF. They are effective in reducing BP, produce a sustained natriuretic and diuretic action, may be used in multidrug regimens, and are more affordable than other antihypertensive agents.[1]

Loop Diuretics

Loop diuretics are reserved for patients with severe heart failure or acute volume overload. Loop diuretics produce greater diuresis than thiazides, are effective in the setting of renal impairment, and have linear dose-response characteristics that allow escalation to high doses when indicated. It should be noted that brisk diuresis with these agents can reduce cardiac filling pressures, decrease cardiac output, and lower blood pressure. An unexplained rise in BUN should be viewed as a sign of a potentially important reduction in tissue perfusion.

Ace Inhibitors

ACE inhibitors are an effective, well-evidenced therapy for the prevention and treatment of heart failure. ACE inhibitors reduce initial ischemic heart disease events and prevent the development of heart failure among patients with hypertension. Two major trials have evidenced the benefit of ACE inhibitors in patients with CAD

TABLE 1.3. Generic oral antihypertensive drugs

Drug class	Drug	Dose range (mg/day)	Daily doses
ACE-I	Benazepril	10–40	1
	Captopril	25–100	2
	Enalopril	5–40	1–2
	Fosinopril	10–40	1
	Lisinopril	10–40	1
	Moexipril	7.5–30	1
	Quinapril	10–80	1
Aldosterone receptor blockers	Spironolactone	25–50	1
Beta and alpha blockers	Carvedilol	12.5–50	2
	Labetalol	200–800	2
Beta blockers	Atenolol	25–100	1
	Betaxolol	5–20	1
	Bisoprolol	2.5–10	1
	Metoprolol	50–100	2
	Metoprolol XL	50–100	1
	Nadolol	40–120	1
	Propranolol	40–160	2
	Propranolol LA	60–180	1
	Timolol	20–40	2
Calcium channel blockers (CCBs) dihydropyridines	Nicardipine SR	60–120	2
	Nifedipine	30–60	1
Loop diuretics	Bumetanide	0.5–2.5	2
	Furosemide	20–80	2
	Torsemide	2.5–10	1
Thiazide diuretics	Chlorothiazide	125–500	1–2
	Chlorthalidone	12.5–25	1
	Hydrochlorothiazide	12.5–50	1
	Indapamide	1.25–2.5	1
	Metolazone	0.5–1.0	1

Adapted from JNC 7 Express. The Seventh Report of the Joint National Committee on P1revention, Detection, Evaluation and Treatment of High Blood Pressure. May 2003. NIH Publication 1No. 03–5233. http:www. nhlbi.nih.gov/guidelines/hypertension/jncintro.htm.

without LV dysfunction or heart failure. The HOPE trial showed a 22% reduction in the combined endpoint of cardiovascular death, MI, or stroke in patients with known CAD or multiple CVD risk factors treated with ramipril 10 mg/day.[20] Similarly, the EUROPA trial showed a 20% relative risk reduction in the composite endpoint of cardiovascular death, MI, or cardiac arrest among patients treated with perindopril vs. placebo.[21]

The benefit of ACE inhibitors for patients with systolic heart failure is well established. In patients with asymptomatic left ventricular dysfunction, ACE inhibitors preserve cardiac function and decrease progression to overt heart failure. In patients with established systolic heart failure, ACE inhibitors increase cardiac output, diminish congestive symptoms by venodilation, reduce progressive cardiac dysfunction, and decrease cardiovascular mortality.[22] These benefits may be attributed to the ability of ACE inhibitors to reduced ventricular remodeling and LV dysfunction following myocardial infarction. In the Acute Infarction Ramipril Efficacy (AIRE) trial, ramipril administered for 3–7 days after MI reduced the relative mortality risk by 41% in hypertensive subjects with LV dysfunction in the post-MI period.[23] The subsequent ATLAS study proved the reduction in mortality is dose dependant, with increased doses improving survival.[24]

The benefit of ACE inhibitors in patients with diastolic dysfunction is less clear. It is known that these agents decrease after load and promote regression of left ventricular hypertrophy, theoretically improving diastolic dysfunction. An additional potential benefit is the reduction of myocardial stiffness through decreased local angiotensin II production. Further studies are needed to investigate long-term clinical outcomes in diastolic heart failure.

When initiating therapy, ACE inhibitors should be started at low doses to reduce the likelihood of hypotension or azotemia. If tolerated, the dose is gradually increased to relatively high maintenance doses used in successful trials (Captopril 50 mg TID; Enalapril 10 mg BID; Lisinopril 35 mg QD; Quinapril 5 mg BID).[24]

Angiotensin Receptor Blockers

Angiotensin II receptor blockers (ARBs) have been shown to reduce the incidence or severity of ischemic heart disease events, renal failure, and cerebrovascular events in patients with hypertension. In the primary prevention of cardiovascular disease, they have similar efficacy to CCBs (amlodipine) as demonstrated in the VALUE study.[25]

In patients with heart failure, ARBs are equally or slightly less effective than ACE inhibitors.[26] The Candesartan in Heart failure: Assessment of Reduction in Mortality and morbidity (CHARM) program showed the use of Candesartan in heart failure patients intolerant of ACE inhibitors resulted in a significant reduction in the primary composite end point of cardiovascular death and hospital readmission for HF.[27] Based on the available data, ARBs are considered an appropriate therapy in heart failure patients who are unable to take ACE inhibitors.

Beta Blockers

Beta blockers are a diverse class of antihypertensive drugs with varied effects on cardiac conduction, cardiac contractility, and blood vessel resistance. The negative ionotopic and chronotropic effects of these agents reduce angina and ischemia in addition to lowering blood pressure. While the evidence of cardio protection from beta blockers in the primary prevention of CVD is weak, their benefit in patients with angina, myocardial ischemia, or LV dysfunction is well established.[17] In patients with systolic heart failure, multiple clinical trials show that the beta blockers such as bisoprolol, metoprolol, and carvedilol improve overall and event-free survival. The Metoprolol XL Randomized Intervention Trial in Heart failure (MERIT-HF) was stopped prematurely when preliminary analysis showed a 34% reduction in mortality among NYHA class II-IV HF patients treated with metoprolol compared to placebo.[28] When compared directly, carvedilol was more effective than metoprolol XL in reducing mortality in patients with heart failure. The Carvedilol or Metoprolol European Trial (COMET) demonstrated a 17% greater mortality reduction with carvedilol compared to metoprolol XL at mean daily doses of 42 mg and 85mg.[29] The mechanism of increased survival was not established but may be related to the alpha blocking properties of carvedilol. In patients with diastolic dysfunction, beta blockers provide benefit by slowing the heart rate to increase left atrial emptying, reducing myocardial oxygen demand, and lowering blood pressure to help reverse left ventricular hypertrophy.[9]

The improved survival of heart failure patients treated with beta blocker therapy appears additive to that induced by ACE inhibitors. Therefore, beta blocker therapy is indicated in patients with NYHA class II-IV heart failure already on an ACE inhibitor and diuretics even in the absence of hypertension. Evidence suggests that the benefits of beta blockers are dose dependant, so low initial doses should be advanced to target doses or until limited by side effects. Target doses are carvedilol 25 mg BID (50 mg BID in patients >85 kg), metoprolol 50–75 mg BID, metoprolol XR 100–200 mg/day, and bisoprolol 5–10 mg once daily.

Aldosterone Receptor Agonists

Aldosterone agonists have not been evaluated for the prevention of cardiovascular disease in hypertensive patients without

LV dysfunction. Studies show benefit as adjunctive therapy for the treatment of hypertension in patients with heart failure. The RALES trial showed a 30% reduction in total mortality among NYHA stage III heart failure patients treated with spironolactone in addition to standard HF therapy.[30] Similar survival benefit was shown with the selective aldosterone inhibitor eplerone in the Eplerenone Post-acute myocardial infarction HEart failure efficacy and SUrvival Study (EPHESUS). In EPHESUS patients with LV dysfunction after MI treated with eplerenone had lower blood pressure and reduced mortality.[31] While heart failure patients with hypertension were not specifically evaluated, the improvement in relative risk with eplerenone was greatest among patents with HF and a history of hypertension. The survival may be related to lower arrhythmic mortality from an elevation in the serum potassium concentration or prevention of the toxic effect of hyperaldosteronism on the heart.

Medications to Avoid

Several classes of drugs should be avoided in patients with heart failure. Nondihydropyridine CCBs such as diltiazem and verapamil are ill advised because their negative inotropic properties may worsen HF symptoms. The dihydropyridine CCB amlodipine, however, appeared to be safe in patients with severe systolic HF in the Prospective Randomized Amlodipine Survival Evaluation (PRAISE) trial.[32] Clonidine is an effective antihypertensive agent but a similar agent, moxonidine, was associated with increased mortality in patients with HF, so both are contraindicated. Finally, alpha blockers should be avoided or used as a last result in patients with heart failure. In the ALLHAT trial, the doxazosin arm was halted due to a twofold increase in relative risk of developing HF when compared with chlorthalidone treatment.[18]

References
1. Chobanian AV, Bakris GI, Black HR, Cushman WC, Green LA, Izzo JL Jr, Jones DW, Materson BJ, Oparil S, Wright JT, Rocella EJ. Joint National Committee on Prevention, Detection, Evaluation, and Treatment of High Blood Pressure; National Heart, Lung, and Blood Institute; National High Blood Pressure Education Program Coordinating Committee. Seventh Report of the Joint National Committee on Prevention, Detection, Evaluation, and Treatment of High Blood Pressure. Hypertension 2003; 42: 1206–1252.
2. Vasan RS, Beiser A, Seshadri S, Larson MG, Kannel WB, D'Agostino RB, Levy D. Residual lifetime risk for developing hypertension in middle-aged women and men: The Framingham Heart Study. J Am Med Assoc 2002; 287: 1003–1010.

3. SHEP Cooperative Research Group. Prevention of stroke by antihypertensive drug treatment in older persons with isolated systolic hypertension. Final results of the Systolic Hypertension in the Elderly Program (SHEP). J Am Med Assoc 1991; 265: 3255–3264.

4. Rosendorff C, Black HR, Cannon CP, Gersh BJ, Gore J, Izzo JL, Jr, Kaplan NM, O'Connor CM, O'Gara PT, Oparil S. Treatment of Hypertension in the Prevention and Management of Ischemic Heart Disease: A Scientific Statement From the American Heart Association Council for High Blood Pressure Research and the Councils on Clinical Cardiology and Epidemiology and Prevention. Circulation 2007; 115: 2761–2788.

5. Levy D, Larson MG, Vasan RS, Kannel WB, Ho KK. The progression from hypertension to congestive heart failure. J Am Med Assoc 1996; 275: 1557–1562.

6. Forette F, Seux ML, Staessen JA, et al. Prevention of dementia in randomized double-blind placebo-controlled Systolic Hypertension in Europe (Syst-Eur) trial. Lancet 1998; 352: 1347–1351.

7. Lewington S, Clarke R, Qizilbash N, Peto R, Collins R. Age-specific relevance of usual blood pressure to vascular mortality: A meta-analysis of individual data for one million adults in 61 prospective studies. Lancet 2002; 360: 1903–1913.

8. Sheps SG, Roccella EJ. Reflections on the sixth report of the Joint National Committee on prevention, detection, evaluation, and treatment of high blood pressure. Curr Hypertens Rep 1999; 1: 342–345.

9. Bonow, RO, Udelson, JE. Left ventricular diastolic dysfunction as a cause of congestive heart failure. Mechanisms and management. Ann Intern Med 1992; 117: 502.

10. Neal B, MacMahon S, Chapman N. Effects of ACE inhibitors, calcium antagonists, and other blood-pressure-lowering drugs: Results of prospectively designed overviews of randomized trials. Blood Pressure Lowering Treatment Trialists' Collaboration. Lancet 2000; 356: 1955–1964.

11. O'Rorke JE, Richardson WS. Evidence based management of hypertension: What to do when blood pressure is difficult to control. Br Med J 2001; 322: 1229–1232.

12. He J, Whelton PK, Appel LJ, Charleston J, Klag MJ. Long-term effects of weight loss and dietary sodium reduction on incidence of hypertension. Hypertension 2000; 35: 544–549.

13. The Trials of Hypertension Prevention Collaborative Research Group. Effects of weight loss and sodium reduction intervention on blood pressure and hypertension incidence in overweight people with high-normal blood pressure. The Trials of Hypertension Prevention, phase II. Arch Intern Med 1997; 157: 657–667.

14. Sacks FM, Svetkey LP, Vollmer WM, et al. Effects on blood pressure of reduced dietary sodium and the Dietary Approaches to Stop Hypertension (DASH) diet. DASH-Sodium Collaborative Research Group. N Engl J Med 2001; 344: 3–10.

15. Whelton SP, Chin A, Xin X, He J. Effect of aerobic exercise on blood pressure: A meta-analysis of randomized, controlled trials. Ann Intern Med 2002; 136: 493–503.

16. Specchia G, De Servi S, Scire A, Assandri J, Berzuini C, Angoli L, La Rovere MT, Cobelli F. Interaction between exercise training and ejection fraction in predicting prognosis after a first myocardial infarction. Circulation 1996; 94: 978–982.

17. Wang JG, Staessen JA. Benefits of antihypertensive pharmacologic therapy and blood pressure reduction in outcome trials. J Clin Hypertens (Greenwich) 2003; 5: 66–75.

18. ALLHAT Officers and Coordinators for the ALLHAT Collaborative Research Group. Major outcomes in high-risk hypertensive patients randomized to angiotensin converting enzyme inhibitor or calcium channel blocker vs diuretic: The Antihypertensive and Lipid-Lowering Treatment to Prevent Heart Attack Trial (ALLHAT). J Am Med Assoc 2002; 288: 2981–2997.

19. Dahlof B, Devereux RB, Kjeldsen SE, et al. Cardiovascular morbidity and mortality in the Losartan Intervention For Endpoint reduction in hypertension study (LIFE): A randomized trial against atenolol. Lancet 2002; 359: 995–1003.

20. Yusuf S, Sleight P, Pogue J, Bosch J, Davies R, Dagenais G. Effects of an angiotensin-converting-enzyme inhibitor, ramipril, on cardiovascular events in high-risk patients: The Heart Outcomes Prevention Evaluation Study. N Engl J Med 2000; 342: 145–153.

21. Fox KM. EURopean trial On reduction of cardiac events with Perindopril in stable coronary Artery disease Investigators. Efficacy of perindopril in reduction of cardiovascular events among patients with stable coronary artery disease: Randomised, double-blind, placebo-controlled, multicenter trial (the EUROPA study). Lancet 2003; 362: 782–788.

22. SOLVD Investigators. Effect of enalapril on survival in patients with reduced left ventricular ejection fractions and congestive heart failure. N Engl J Med 1991; 325: 293.

23. Acute Infarction Ramipril Efficacy (AIRE) Study Investigators. Effect of ramipril on mortality and morbidity of survivors of acute myocardial infarction with clinical evidence of heart failure. Lancet 1993; 342: 821–828.

24. Packer M, Poole-Wilson PA, Armstrong PW, Cleland JG, Horowitz JD, Massie BM, Ryden L, Thygesen K, Uretsky BF. ATLAS Study Group. Comparative effects of low and high doses of the angiotensin-converting enzyme inhibitor, lisinopril, on morbidity and mortality in chronic heart failure. Circulation 1999; 100: 2312–2318.

25. Julius S, Kjeldsen SE, Weber M, Brunner HR, Ekman S, Hansson L, Hua T, Laragh J, McInnes GT, Mitchell L, Plat F, Schork A, Smith B, Zanchetti A. VALUE Trial Group. Outcomes in hypertensive patients at high cardiovascular risk treated with regimens based on valsartan or amlodipine: The VALUE randomised trial. Lancet 2004; 363: 2022–2031.

26. Pfeffer MA, McMurray JJ, Velazquez EJ, Rouleau JL, Kober L, Maggioni AP, Solomon SD, Swedberg K, Van de Werf F, White H, Leimberger JD, Henis M, Edwards S, Zelenkofske S, Sellers MA, Califf

RM. Valsartan in Acute Myocardial Infarction Trial Investigators. Valsartan, captopril, or both in myocardial infarction complicated by heart failure, left ventricular dysfunction, or both. N Engl J Med 2003; 349; 1893–1906

27. Granger CB, McMurray JJ, Yusuf S, Held P, Michelson EL, Olofsson B, Ostergren J, Pfeffer MA, Swedberg K. CHARM Investigators and Committees. Effects of candesartan in patients with chronic heart failure and reduced left ventricular systolic function intolerant to angiotensin-converting-enzyme inhibitors: The CHARM-Alternative trial. Lancet 2003; 362: 772–776.

28. MERIT-HF Study Group. Effect of metoprolol CR/XL in chronic heart failure: Metoprolol CR/XL Randomized Intervention Trial in Congestive Heart Failure (MERIT-HF). Lancet 1999; 353: 2001–2007.

29. Poole-Wilson PA, Swedberg K, Cleland JG, Di Lenarda A, Hanrath P, Komajda M, Lubsen J, Lutiger B, Metra M, Remme WJ, Torp-Pedersen C, Scherhag A, Skene A. Carvedilol Or Metoprolol European Trial Investigators. Comparison of carvedilol and metoprolol on clinical outcomes in patients with chronic heart failure in the Carvedilol Or Metoprolol European Trial (COMET): Randomised controlled trial. Lancet 2003; 362: 7–13.

30. Pitt B, Zannad F, Remme WJ, Cody R, Castaigne A, Perez A, Palensky J, Wittes J. Randomized Aldactone Evaluation Study Investigators (RALES). The effect of spironolactone on morbidity and mortality in patients with severe heart failure. N Engl J Med 1999; 341: 709–717.

31. Pitt B, Remme W, Zannad F, Neaton J, Martinez F, Roniker B, Bittman R, Hurley S, Kleiman J, Gatlin M. Eplerenone Post-Acute Myocardial Infarction Heart Failure Efficacy and Survival Study Investigators. Eplerenone, a selective aldosterone blocker, in patients with left ventricular dysfunction after myocardial infarction. (EPHESUS) N Engl J Med 2003; 348: 1309–1321.

32. O'Connor CM, Carson PE, Miller AB, Pressler ML, Belkin RN, Neuberg GW, Frid DJ, Cropp AB, Anderson S, Wertheimer JH, DeMets DL. Effect of amlodipine on mode of death among patients with advanced heart failure in the PRAISE trial: Prospective randomized amlodipine survival evaluation. Am J Cardiol 1998; 82: 881–887.

Chapter 2
Coronary Artery Disease Prevention

Saadia Sherazi and Robert Block

Atherosclerotic cardiovascular disease is the leading cause of death in both men and women in the United States. It is associated with significant health burden causing premature disability and mortality. Data from the National Health and Nutrition Survey (NHANES) suggests that 3.7 million persons in the United States are living with coronary heart disease (CHD).[1] The prevalence of disease in men and women increases with advancing age. Although cardiovascular mortality has declined since 1975, this trend has slowed since 1990.[2–7] Advances in medical therapy have contributed approximately 45% to this reduction with the remaining 55% due to risk factor reduction. The risk factors most successfully modified have been smoking, hypertension, and hypercholestrolemia.[2,3]

The primary prevention of coronary artery disease aims to reduce the risk of disease in subjects free of diagnosed disease. One of the keys to reducing the burden of heart disease nation-wide is to focus attention on the identification of risk factors and subsequently their modification. Evidence that most cardiovascular disease (CVD) is preventable led to the development of the American Heart Association's initial "Guide to the Primary Prevention of Cardiovascular Disease" in 1996 and an updated version in 2002.[8,9] According to this consensus statement, the following factors are modifiable and should be evaluated in all adults: smoking, hypertension, diet, dyslipidemia, physical inactivity, obesity, and diabetes mellitus (considered a CHD risk equivalent).

J.D. Bisognano et al. (eds.), *Manual of Heart Failure Management*, DOI: 10.1007/978-1-84882-185-9_2, © Springer-Verlag London Limited 2009

Patients with established coronary artery disease require secondary prevention and tend to have a higher risk of subsequent myocardial infarction, stroke, and death from CVD than those without coronary disease. Patients with diagnosed noncoronary atherosclerotic disease, multiple risk factors that confer a 10-year risk of CHD of ≥20%, diabetes, and chronic kidney disease with serum creatinine concentration exceeding 1.5 mg/mL are considered to have a CHD risk equivalent. Intensive risk factor modification for all patients in the categories described above is recommended by Adult Treatment Panel III (ATP III) and the 2006 ACC/AHA guidelines on secondary prevention.[10,11]

SMOKING

Cigarette smoking is associated with increased incidence and mortality from CVD.[2] Numerous studies have shown the impact of smoking cessation and risk reduction from coronary artery disease.[12] The risk of myocardial infarction and death from coronary artery disease is reduced to one-half after 1 year of smoking cessation with the risk approaching that of nonsmokers after several years of quitting smoking.[13] The US Public Health Service released a clinical practice guideline in 2000 on Treating Tobacco Use and Dependence that summarizes scientific research on techniques for effective cessation of cigarette smoking.[14] The Guideline recommends that smokers be offered both counseling and medications. Self-help materials were not found to be particularly effective. Individual counseling and group counseling, however, were found to increase the success rates for smoking cessation. Social support from healthcare providers, family, friends, and other community members increases the success rate of abstinence from smoking.

HYPERTENSION

Higher relative systolic and diastolic blood pressures are associated with coronary artery disease.[15] In addition, isolated systolic hypertension is now a well-established coronary risk factor.[16] The recommendations of the Seventh Joint National Committee (JNC7) provide guidelines for the treatment of patients with hypertension.[17] The evidences that led to these guidelines support dividing patients into subgroups according to the level of blood pressure and comorbidities. The guidelines support maintaining blood pressure <140/90 mmHg or <130/80 mmHg if the patient has diabetes or proteinuric chronic kidney disease. Life style modifications including weight loss, exercise, and salt restriction have shown to prevent the development of hypertension in individuals with prehypertension (blood pressure systolic 120–139 mmHg).

In contrast, a lack of data exists to support the use of antihypertensive agents in prehypertension subjects. The choice of antihypertensive agent is optimally determined by the risk factor profile and comorbidities and is addressed elsewhere in this book.

DYSLIPIDEMIA

Lipoprotein disorders are considered significant risk factors for both coronary artery disease and other atherosclerotic vascular diseases. Evidence from randomized controlled trials strongly supports the treatment of all patients with CAD with lipid lowering agents to reduce their risk of subsequent events.[18–20] This evidence extends to patients with a CAD risk equivalent (peripheral vascular disease, diabetes mellitus, and patients with an absolute risk of coronary events ≥20%). and to some subjects without CAD or elevated cholesterol.[21–23] Lipid lowering strategies should focus beyond targeting LDL-C, as triglycerides, non-high density (HDL) cholesterol, and HDL cholesterol are also of significant importance. Disorders of lipoprotein metabolism can be broadly divided into two categories: primary disorders, which are inherited, and secondary disorders resulting from another condition. The list of secondary causes includes hypothyroidism, diabetes mellitus, renal disease, alcohol, and numerous drugs that should be considered in the evaluation of patients presenting with a lipoprotein disorder.

Primary Prevention

The most important step involved in lipid management in subjects in the realm of primary prevention of coronary artery disease involves a careful risk assessment with subsequent selection of the appropriate therapy. As mentioned, strong evidence supports the use of both pharmacological and nonpharmacological measures to treat lipid disorders in the primary prevention of CAD. Recently, Ford and Colleagues reported results after 10 years of follow up of the West of Scotland Coronary Prevention Study (WOSCOPS) that include more than 90% of the original trial survivors.[24] They found a statistically significant difference in death from CHD or nonfatal myocardial with a rate of 10.3% in the group originally assigned to placebo and 8.6% in the group originally assigned to pravastatin. This study had originally shown a reduction in coronary mortality by lowering serum cholesterol with pravastatin in middle-aged men with serum LDL-cholesterol concentrations above 155 milligrams per deciliter (mg/dL).[23] The benefits were replicated in the Air Force/Texas Coronary Atherosclerosis Prevention Study (AFCAPS/TexCAPS) in which the use of lovastatin was associated with reduced coronary events in low risk men and women without prior evidence of coronary artery disease.[21] The Anglo-Scandinavian Cardiac Outcomes Trial-Lipid Lowering Arm (ASCOT-LLA) showed similar benefit on the primary endpoint of myocardial infarction and fatal CHD in patients receiving atorvastatin.[22]

Secondary Prevention
The major secondary prevention trials using statin therapy are summarized in Table 2.1. Strong evidence from several trials support current recommendations and these include the Scandinavian Simvastatin Survival Study (4S) in which a 30% reduction in cerebrovascular events in patients with coronary artery disease and elevated LDL was shown.[20] The Cholesterol And Recurrent Events (CARE) study and the Long-term Intervention with Pravastatin in Ischemic Disease (LIPID) study revealed benefit from the use of lipid lowering therapy in patients with CAD and mild to moderately elevated LDL level.[18,19] The results from numerous clinical trials have led to the development of current guidelines aiming for LDL-C less than 100 mg/dL and even less than 70 mg/dL in high risk patients.[10,11]

Drug Therapy for Lipid Modification

3-Hydroxy-3-Methylglutaryl Coenzyme A (HMG CoA) Reductase Inhibitors
The development of 3-hydroxy-3-methylglutaryl coenzyme A (HMG CoA) reductase inhibitors, or statins, led to the most important advances in the management of CVD. Statins are the most commonly used agents for the treatment of hypercholesterolemia because of their safety, efficacy, and tolerability. Statins are highly effective in reducing LDL-C by inhibiting the rate-limiting step in cholesterol synthesis. Triglyceride lowering tends to be directly proportional to the baseline triglyceride level and to the LDL-lowering potency of the drug. On average, statins tend to increase HDL-C by 5–10% and this effect is not dose dependent. There are six statins currently available: lovastatin, pravastatin, simvastatin, fluvastatin, atorvastatin, and rosuvastatin. Interestingly, clinical benefits associated with statins are evident early in the course of lipid-lowering therapy before angiographic plaque regression has occurred.[32] In WOSCOPS, the CHD event rate in pravastatin treated patients was not related to the magnitude of LDL cholesterol level lowering.[23] These analyses suggest that nonlipid mechanisms of statins may contribute to their ability to reduce cardiovascular events and explain the early clinical benefit in WOSCOPS and several other studies.[21,32–36] In addition

TABLE 2.1. Secondary prevention trials

Clinical trials	Intervention	Outcome/reduction
The Coronary Drug Project[25]	Niacin	Reduction in nonfatal MI after 6 years of treatment. Reduction in total mortality after 15 years of follow up[26]
The Program on the Surgical Control of Hyperlipidemias (POSCH)[27]	Partial ileal bypass surgery to reduce LDL-C	35% Relative reduction in fatal CHD and nonfatal MI, with no effect on total mortality
Lipid Research Clinics Coronary Primary Prevention Trial (LRC-CPPT)[28,29]	Cholestyramine	19% Relative reduction in combined fatal CHD and nonfatal MI
Scandinavian Simvastatin Survival Study (4S Trial)[20]	Simvastatin	30% Relative risk reduction in total mortality and 44% reduction in CHD death or MI
Cholesterol and Recurrent Events (CARE) Study[19]	Pravastatin	24% Reduction in relative risk of combined fatal CHD
Long-Term Intervention with Pravastatin in Ischemic Disease Study (LIPID Trial)[18]	Pravastatin	24% Reduction in CHD mortality
		22% Reduction in total mortality
The Heart Protection Study (HPS)[30]	Simvastatin	24% Reduction in major coronary events and 13% reduction in total mortality
The Prospective Study of Pravastatin in the Elderly at Risk (PROSPER)[31]	Pravastain	15% Reduction in cardiovascular end points
The Anglo-Scandinavian Cardiac Outcomes Trial Lipid Lowering Arm (ASCOTT-LLA)[22]	Atorvastatin	36% Relative risk reduction

to lowering low-density lipoprotein cholesterol, statin therapy appears to exert beneficial pleiotropic effects on the atherosclerotic process including endothelial function,[37–39] inflammation,[40] plaque stability,[41,42] and thrombus formation.[43–45] Laufs et al.

have shown that the inhibition of HMG CoA reductase in vascular endothelial cells leads to up-regulation of endothelial cell NO synthase (ecNOS) expression and activity through effects on oxidized LDL.[46] This effect of HMG CoA reductase inhibitors on ecNOS expression contributes to the restoration of endothelial function beyond that achieved by reduction in serum cholesterol levels alone. As stated above, many studies have shown improvements in endothelial function with statin therapy and this improvement has been shown in patients with and without coronary artery disease.[37–39,47] In fact, a recent study has shown improvement in endothelial function occurring as early as 3 days with statin therapy.[48] Statins are generally well tolerated but some patients develop increased transaminase levels, fatigue, or myalgias. The etiology of myalgias ranges from no pathophysiologic findings to mild myositis and rhabdomyolysis.[18–20] Risk factors for statin myopathy that should be kept in mind include advanced age, renal insufficiency, frailty, occult hypothyroidism, and female gender.

Cholesterol Absorption Inhibitors

Ezetimibe is available as the first cholesterol absorption inhibitor that acts at the intestinal brush border. Although it has been shown to lower LDL cholesterol alone and in combination with a statin, no cardiovascular outcome data is available.[49] The combination of simvastatin plus ezetimibe as one drug is commercially available. Recent study showed that in patients with familial hypercholesterolemia, combined therapy with ezetimibe and simvastatin did not result in a significant difference in changes in intima-media thickness, as compared with simvastatin alone, despite decreases in levels of LDL cholesterol.[50] Until IMPROVE-IT study is completed, the potential benefits in reducing CVD outcomes of the combination of these two drugs will be unknown.[51] In the meantime, the recommendations are to: First, achieve targets for levels of LDL and HDL cholesterol with the use of statins plus drugs that have shown clinical benefits when added to statins. Second, use ezetimibe only in patients who, despite the above-mentioned therapy, do not achieve their individual targets.[52]

Bile Acid Sequestrants (Resins)

Cholestyramine and Colestipol are the classic agents included in this group of lipid lowering agents. Their clinical use, however, has been limited by the somewhat unsavory formulations that patients need to ingest. Colesevalam is a newer agent with somewhat better compliance as, due to its molecular structure, it more effectively binds to bile acids. Resins are effective at lowering LDL-C and have a minimal effect of raising HDL-C. Their use is also supported by results from clinical trials demonstrating a reduction in cardiovascular events.[28,29] Due to the protential side effects that include bloating and constipation, resins are often best reserved for use in patients intolerant of other cholesterol-lowering agents. Moreover, their use should be avoided in patients with high triglycerdies due to the fact that inhibiting cholesterol absorption can lead to a compensatory increase in hepatic production of VLDL.

Fibric Acid Derivatives (Fibrates)

This group includes clofibrate, gemfibrozil, fenofibrate, and bezafibrate. Their main role is in triglyceride lowering (up to 40%), with a modest effect on raising HDL (up to 20%) and more neutral effects on altering levels of LDL-C.[53] As a group, fibrates have demonstrated in clinical trials an ability to reduce cardiovascular events with perhaps the strongest effect noted with gemfibrozil in the Veterans Affairs High-Density Lipoprotein Cholesterol Intervention Trial (VA-HIT).[54] In this study, patients with low HDL-C randomized to gemfibrozil had a 22% reduction in risk of cardiovascular death, with an approximate 3% reduction for every 1% increase in HDL-C. These drugs are useful as first line treatment in patients with triglycerides more than 500 mg/dL. They can also be useful in patients with isolated low HDL as they increase HDL modestly. Fibrates can be a particularly useful component in the strategy for attacking the increased risk of cardiovascular events in patients with insulin resistance, metabolic syndrome, or type 2 diabetes.[53] The most common side effect is dyspepsia.

Nicotinic Acid (Niacin)

Nicotinic acid or niacin is a B-complex vitamin that has been used for lowering triglycerides and LDL and increasing HDL. Niacin is the pharmaceutical agent with the strongest HDL raising effects and its efficacy in reducing non-fatal MI and total mortality was demonstrated in the Coronary Drug Project.[25] The clinical use of niacin can be limited by its side effects of severe flushing but when patients concomitantly take aspirin prior to dosing, take it with a snack and avoid drinking hot-liquids at the time of dosing, the drug can be very well tolerated. This side effect can also be minimized with the use of a sustained-release formulation. An additional side effect encountered can be the elevation of uric acid levels and in some patients this can lead to gout. A clinical scenario in which niacin can be particularly effective is when a patient has the metabolic syndrome/insulin resistance with elevated triglycerides, low HDL, and elevated non-HDL cholesterol. Due to the beneficial properties of niacin on fatty acid metabolism and VLDL production, it can also be a highly complementary agent when used in combination with a statin.[55]

Omega-3 Fatty Acids
Omega-3 fatty acids are quite potent modulators of lipid metabolism and their clinical use for treating hypertriglyceridemia is supported by strong evidence.[56,57] The omega-3 fatty acids, derived from fish {eicosapentaenoic acid (EPA) and docosapentaenoic acid (DHA)}, have also been demonstrated to reduce the risk of cardiac events in subjects with known coronary artery disease.[56] Although omega-3 fatty acids exert anti-inflammatory and lipid-altering effects, much of the interest in their cardioprevention effects revolves around their potent antiarrhythmic effects.[58] The most commonly used fish oil supplements are over-the-counter and contain approximately 30% EPA + DHA but a pharmaceutical-grade EPA + DHA formulation has also been available in the United States. This concentrated agent is approved at a dose of 4 g/day for treating triglyceride levels of >500 g/dL.

DIET
Substantial evidence from clinical studies has emphatically shown that diet correlates with risk of coronary artery disease.[34,59–63] The list of beneficial foods includes using fruits, vegetables (especially cruciferous vegetables such as broccoli, cauliflower, cabbage, and brussel sprouts), green leafy vegetables, and citrus fruits. The consumption of foods rich in fiber has been associated with a 40–50% reduction in the risk of CHD. Among high fiber diets, cereals are most strongly associated with a reduced risk of myocardial infarction.[61,62] Individuals who consume small to moderate amounts of alcohol have a lower risk of CVD including reduced cardiovascular mortality.[64–66] However, these benefits should be weighed against a potential increase in risk of numerous cancers including those of the liver, esophagus, larynx, colon, and breast.[67–69] Observational studies have demonstrated that the use of fish is associated with lower risk of CHD mortality. As mentioned, the beneficial effects of fish consumption have been ascribed due to n-3 fatty acids, which have also shown in randomized trials of supplements to decrease subsequent CVD.[56] Some uncertainty exists regarding the scientific basis for how foods are protective as most of the data comes from

observational studies where results could have been confounded. For example, people who eat healthier food and consume more fruits and vegetables also may have healthy life styles in ways that can be difficult to measure.

The dietary approach should include a thorough general assessment of the dietary habits of patients by healthcare providers, and suggestions should be provided accordingly. Appropriate recommendations should be individualized and target the specific type of hyperlipidemia. For example, patients with elevated LDL-C benefit from a reduction in their intake of saturated fats and cholesterol, whereas patients with hypertriglyceridemia benefit from reduced intake of simple carbohydrates and overall calories. A formal consultation with a dietician is crucial and should be strongly encouraged in situations when patients require more than minimal education or lifestyle modification. Plant stanols, which are available in the form of spreads and snack bars, can actively reduce absorption of LDL-C and are thus additional weapons in the armamentarium. Soy proteins have been shown to reduce serum cholesterol levels and fish oils, as mentioned above, can reduce triglyceride levels when used in higher doses.

OBESITY

Data from the Framingham Heart Study, Nurse's Health Study, and other studies have shown an association between obesity and CVD.[70–72] Multiple risk factors of atherosclerosis are associated with obesity including hypertension, high cholesterol, insulin resistance, glucose intolerance, low serum HDL cholesterol, and high plasma fibrinogen concentrations. All overweight subjects should undergo a risk assessment and be provided with information about diet, exercise, and behavior modification. It is imperative to understand that health promotion programs focusing behavioral risk factors have been effective among highly educated, fully employed, and highly motivated individuals. This methodology, however, has been more limited in certain high-risk individuals including subjects from rural areas, those in the working class, and the poor. These individuals more often exist in a vicious circle of a higher risk of CHD associated with higher rates of smoking, physical inactivity, psychological stress, and diets higher in saturated fat. These facts underscore the need to understand the limitations that can exist in vulnerable subject groups and to adopt alternative methodologies to improve life styles. One potential strategy is to improve the social environment by providing access to affordable, healthy foods, and recreational facilities.

DIABETES

Among patients with type 1 diabetes mellitus, intensive insulin therapy has shown to decrease fatal and nonfatal cardiovascular events.[73] Cardiovascular events, including nonfatal MI, stroke, or CVD death were reduced to 42% in those patients intensively treated in the Diabetes Complications and Control Trial.[73] There is some controversy to the benefits of tight glycemic control in patients with type 2 diabetes. The United Kingdom Prospective Diabetes Study found no statistical difference in macrovascular disease in the intensive and conventional therapy groups though secondary analyses showed that reducing the HbA1C value by 1% was associated with an 18% reduction in MI.[74]

OTHER DRUG THERAPIES FOR CORONARY ARTERY PREVENTION

Aspirin is a potent therapy for reducing CVD events in adults who are at an increased risk. In a recent meta-analysis, aspirin therapy was associated with a 12% reduction in cardiovascular events in women and a 14% reduction in men but it did increase the incidence of bleeding in both women and men.[75] The United States Preventive Services Task Force (USPSTF) recommends the use of aspirin for primary prevention of coronary disease for men and women whose 5-year risk of a first CHD event is 3% or greater as calculated by the Framingham risk score.[76] The same recommendations are part of primary prevention guidelines for men and women whose 10-year risk of a first CHD event is 10% or greater from the American Heart Association (AHA).[9,77] These guidelines are supported by data from the Antithrombotic Trialists' Collaboration's overview of 195 randomized trials of antiplatelet therapy among 135,000 patients with prior evidence of CVD. Those data revealed a 25% reduction in the risk of subsequent vascular events.[78]

Beta-blockers have been shown to decrease mortality by 20% in patients with prior myocardial infarction and upto 35% in patients with depressed left ventricular systolic function.[79] Considerable experimental and clinical data supports the use of angiotensin-converting enzyme (ACE) inhibitors due to demonstrated anti-atherosclerotic effects that are independent of reductions in blood pressure.[1,80] These benefits of ACE inhibition are likely due to attenuation of the contractile and superoxide-generating effects of angiotensin II and to enhancement of endothelial cell release of nitric oxide secondary to diminished breakdown of bradykinin.

Acknowledgments The project described was supported by Grant Number KL2 RR 024136 from the National Center for Research Resources (NCRR), a component of the National Institutes of Health (NIH) and the NIH Roadmap for Medical Research, and its contents are solely the responsibility of the authors and do not necessarily represent the official view of NCRR or NIH. Information on NCRR is available at http://www.ncrr.nih.gov/. Information on Re-engineering the Clinical Research Enterprise can be obtained from http://nihroadmap.nih.gov/clinicalresearch/overview-translational.asp.

References

1. Al-Mallah MH, Tleyjeh IM, Abdel-Latif AA, et al (2006) Angiotensin-converting enzyme inhibitors in coronary artery disease and preserved left ventricular systolic function: a systematic review and meta analysis of randomized controlled trials. J Am Coll Cardiol 47:1576–1583.

2. Capewell S, Morrison CE, McMurray JJ (1999) Contribution of modern cardiovascular treatment and risk factor changes to the decline in coronary heart disease mortality in Scotland between 1975 and 1994. Heart 81:380–386.

3. Capewell S, Beaglehole R, Seddon M, McMurray J (2000) Explanation for the decline in coronary heart disease mortality rates in Auckland, New Zealand, between 1982 and 1993. Circulation 102:1511–1516.

4. Cooper R, Cutler J, Desvigne-Nickens P, et al (2000) Trends and disparities in coronary heart disease, stroke, and other cardiovascular diseases in the United States: findings of the national conference on cardiovascular disease prevention. Circulation 102:3137–3147.

5. Kuulasmaa K, Tunstall-Pedoe H, Dobson A, et al (2000) Estimation of contribution of changes in classic risk factors to trends in coronary-events rates across the WHO MONICA Project populations. Lancet 355:675–687.

6. McGovern PG, Pankow JS, Shahar E, et al (1996) Recent trends in acute coronary heart disease: mortality, morbidity, medical care, and risk factors. The Minnesota Heart Survey Investigators. N Engl J Med 334:884–890.

7. McGovern PG, Jacobs DR Jr, Shahar E, et al (2001) Trends in acute coronary heart disease mortality, morbidity, and medical care from 1985 through 1997: The Minnesota heart survey. Circulation 104:19–24.

8. Grundy SM, Balady GJ, Criqui MH, et al (1997) Guide to primary prevention of cardiovascular disease. A statement for healthcare professionals from the Task Force on Risk Reduction. American heart Association Science Advisory and Coordination Committee. Circulation 95:2329–2331.

9. Pearson TA, Blair SN, Daniels SR, et al (2002) AHA guidelines for primary prevention of cardiovascular disease and stroke: 2002 Update: Consensus panel guide to comprehensive risk reduction for adult

patients without coronary or other atherosclerotic vascular diseases. American Heart Association Science Advisory and Coordinating Committee. Circulation 106:388–391.

10. Grundy SM, Cleeman JI, Merz CNB, et al (2004) Implication of recent clinical trials for the national cholesterol education program. Adult Treatment Panel III Guidelines. Circulation 110:227–239.

11. Smith SC, Allen J, Blair SN, et al (2006) AHA/ACC guidelines for secondary prevention for patients with coronary and other atherosclerotic vascular disease: 2006 Update: Endorsed by the national heart, lung, and blood institute. Circulation 113:2363–2372.

12. Shinton R, Beevers G (1989) Meta-analysis of relation between cigarette smoking and stroke. Br Med J 298:789–794.

13. Negri E, La Vecchia C, D'Avanzo B, et al (1994) Acute myocardial infarction: associated with time since stopping smoking in Italy. GISSI-EFRIM Investigators. J Epidemiol Community Health 48:129–133.

14. Fiore MC, Bailey WC, Cohen SJ, et al (2000) Treating Tobacco Use and Dependence: Clinical Practice Guideline. Rockville, MD: US Department of Health and Human Services Public Health Service.

15. Kannel WB, Gordon T, Schwartz MJ (1971) Systolic versus diastolic blood pressure and risk of coronary heart disease: The Framingham Study. Am J Cardiol 27:335–345.

16. Wilking SVB, Belanger AJ, Kannel WB, et al (1988) Determinants of isolated systolic blood pressure. J Am Med Assoc 260:3451–3455.

17. Chobanian AV, Bakris GL, Black HR, et al (2003) The Seventh Report of the Joint National Committee on Prevention, Detection, Evaluation, and Treatment of High Blood Pressure: The JNC 7 Report. J Am Med Assoc 289:2560–2572.

18. Long-Term Intervention with Pravastatin in Ischemic Disease (LIPID) Study Group (1998) Prevention of cardiovascular events and death with pravastatin in patients with coronary heart disease and a broad range of initial cholestrol levels. N Engl J Med 339:1349–1357.

19. Sacks FM, Pfeffer MA, Moye L, et al (1996) The effect of pravastatin on coronary events after myocardial infarction in patients with average cholesterol levels. N Engl J Med 335:1001–1009.

20. Scandinavian Simvastatin Survival Study Group (1994) Randomised trial of cholesterol lowering in 4444 patients with coronary heart disease: the Scandinavian Simvastatin Survival Study (4S). Lancet 344:1383–1389.

21. Downs JR, Clearfield M, Weis S, et al (1998) Primary prevention of acute coronary events with lovastatin in men and women with average cholesterol levels: results of AFCAPS/TexCAPS. J Am Med Assoc 279:1615–1622.

22. Sever PS, Dahlof B, Poulter NR, et al (2003) Prevention of coronary and stroke events with atorvastatin in hypertensive patients who have average or lower-than-average cholesterol concentrations, in the Anglo-Scandinavian Cardiac Outcomes Trial-Lipid Lowering Arm (ASCOT-LLA): a multicenter randomized controlled trial. Lancet 361:1149–1158.

23. West of Scotland Coronary Prevention Study Group (1998) Influence of pravastatin and plasma lipids on clinical events in the West of Scotland Coronary Prevention Study (WOSCOPS). Circulation 97:1440–1445.

24. Ford I, Murray H, Packard CJ, et al (2007) Long-term follow-up of the West of Scotland Coronary Prevention Study. N Engl J Med 357:1477–1486.

25. The Coronary Drug Project Research Group (1975) Clofibrate and niacin in coronary heart disease. J Am Med Assoc 231:360–381.

26. Canner P, Berge KG, Wenger NK, et al (1986) Fifteen year mortality in Coronary Drug Project patients: long term benefit with niacin. J Am Coll Cardiol 8:1245–1255.

27. Buchwald H, Varco RL, Matts JP, et al (1990) Effects of partial ileal bypass surgery on mortality and morbidity from coronary heart disease in patients with hypercholesterolemia-report of the program on the surgical control of the hyperlipidemias (POSCH). N Engl Med 323:946–955.

28. Lipid Research Clinics Program (1984) The Lipid Research Clinics Coronary Primary Prevention Trial results 1. Reduction in incidence of coronary heart disease. J Am Med Assoc 251:351–364.

29. Lipid Research Clinics Program (1984) The Lipid Research Clinics Coronary Primary Prevention Trial results 2. The relationship of reduction in incidence of coronary heart disease to cholesterol lowering. J Am Med Assoc 251:365–374.

30. Heart Protection Study Collaborative Group (2002) MRC/BHF Heart Protection Study of cholesterol lowering with simvastatin in 20,536 high-risk individuals: a randomized placebo-controlled trial. Lancet 360:7–22.

31. Shepherd J, Blauw GJ, Murphy MB, et al (2002) Pravastatin in elderly individuals at risk of vascular disease (PROSPER): a randomized controlled trial. Lancet 360:1623–1630.

32. Jukema JW, Bruschke AVG, Van Boven AJ, et al (1995) Effects of lipid lowering by pravastatin on progression and regression of coronary artery disease in symptomatic men with normal to moderately elevated serum cholesterol levels: the Regression Growth Evaluation Statin Study (REGRESS). Circulation 91:2528–2540.

33. Sacks FM, Pfeffer MA, Moye LA, et al (1998) The effect of pravastatin on coronary events in patients with average cholesterol levels. Circulation 97:1446–1452.

34. Schwartz GG, Olsson AG, Ezekowitz MD, et al (2001) Effects of atorvastatin on early recurrent ischemic events in acute coronary syndromes. The MIRACL Study: a randomized controlled trial. J Am Med Assoc 285:1711–1718.

35. Shepherd J, Cobb SM, Ford I, et al (1995) Prevention of coronary heart disease with pravastatin in men with hypercholesterolemia. N Engl J Med 333:1301–1307.

36. The Pravastatin Multinational Study Group for Cardiac Risks Patients (1993) Effects of pravastatin in patients with serum total cholesterol levels from 5.2 to 7.8 mmol/Liter (200 to 300 mg/dl) plus two additional atherosclerotic risk factors. Am J Cardiol 72:1031–1037.

37. Anderson TJ, Meredith IT, Yeung AC, et al (1995) The effect of cholesterol-lowering and antioxidant therapy on endothelium-dependent coronary vasomotion. N Engl J Med 332:488–493.

38. Egashira K, Hirooka Y, Kai H, et al (1994) Reduction in serum cholesterol with pravastatin improves endothelium-dependent coronary vasomotion in patients with hypercholesterolemia. Circulation 89:2519–2524.

39. Treasure CB, Klein JL, Weintraub WS, et al (1995) Beneficial effects of cholesterol-lowering therapy on the coronary endothelium in patients with coronary artery disease. N Engl J Med 332:481–487.

40. Kimura M, Kurose I, Russell J, et al (1997) Effect of fluvastatin on leukocyte-endothelial cell adhesion in hypercholesterolemic rats. Arterioscler Thromb Vasc Biol 17:1521–1526.

41. Shiomi M, Ito T, Tsukada T, et al (1995) Reduction of serum cholesterol levels alters lesional composition of atherosclerotic plaques: effect of pravastatin sodium on atherosclerosis in mature WHHL rabbits. Arterioscler Thromb Vasc Biol 15:1938–1944.

42. Williams JK, Sukhova GK, Herrington DM, et al (1998) Pravastatin has cholesterol lowering independent effects on the artery wall of atherosclerotic monkeys. J Am Coll Cariol 31:684–691.

43. Beigel Y, Fuchs J, Snir M, et al (1991) Lovastatin therapy in hypercholesterolemia: effect on fibrinogen, hemorrheologic parameters, platelet activity and red blood cell morphology. J Clin Pharmacol 31:512–517.

44. Lacoste L, Lam JY, Hung J, et al (1995) Hyperlipidemia and coronary disease. Correction of the increased thrombogenic potential with cholesterol reduction. Circulation 92:3172–3177.

45. Mayer J, Eller T, Brauer P, et al (1992) Effects of long-term treatment with lovastatin on the clotting system and blood platelets. Ann Hematol 64:196–201.

46. Laufs U, La Fata V, Plutzky J (1998) Upregulation of endothelial nitric oxide synthase by HMG CoA reductase inhibitors. Circulation 97:1129–1135.

47. Vogel RA (1999) Cholesterol lowering and endothelial function. Am J Med 107:479–487.

48. Tsunekawa T, Hayashi T, Kano H, et al (2001) Cerivastatin, a Hydroxymethylglutaryl Coenzyme A reductase inhibitor, improves endothelial function in elderly diabetic patients within 3 days. Circulation 104:376–379.

49. Davidson MH, McGarry T, Bettis R, et al (2002) Ezetimibe coadministered with simvastatin in patients with primary hypercholesterolemia. J Am Coll Cardiol 40:2125–2134.

50. Kastelein JJP, Akdim F, Stroes E, et al (2008) Simvastatin with or without Ezetimibe in Familial Hypercholesterolemia. N Engl J Med 358:1431–1443.

51. Strony J (2008) IMPROVE-IT: examining outcomes in subjects with acute coronary syndrome:Vytorin (Ezetimibe/Simvastatin) vs Simvastatin (Study P04103). http://clinicaltrials.gov/show/NCT00202878. Accessed 11 April 2008.

52. Greg Brown B, Taylor AJ (2008) Does ENHANCE diminish confidence in lowering LDL or in ezetimibe? N Engl J Med 358:1504–1507.

53. Steiner G (2004) Fibrates in the metabolic syndrome and in diabetes. Endocrinol Metab Clin North Am 33:545–555.

54. Rubins HB, Robins SJ, Collins D, et al (1999) Gemfibrozil for the secondary prevention of coronary heart disease in men with low levels of high-density lipoprotein cholesterol. N Engl J Med 341:410–418.

55. Levy D, Pearson TA (2005) Combination niacin and statin therapy in primary and secondary prevention of cardiovascular disease. Clin Cardiol 28:317–320.

56. GISSI-Prevenzione Investigators (1999) Dietary supplementation with n-3 polyunsaturated fatty acids and vitamin E after myocardial infarction; results of the GISSI-Prevenzione trial. Lancet 354:447–455.

57. Hooper L, Thompson RL, Harrison RA, et al (2004) Omega 3 fatty acids for prevention and treatment of cardiovascular disease. Cochrane Database Syst Rev, CD003177.

58. Kris-Etherton PM, Harris WS, Appel LJ (2002) Fish consumption, fish oil, omega-3 fatty acids, and cardiovascular disease. Circulation 106:2747–2757.

59. Ascherio A, Rimm EB, Hernan MA, et al (1998) Intake of potassium, magnesium, calcium, and fiber and risk of stroke among US men. Circulation 98:1198–1204.

60. Gillman MW, Cupples LA, Gagnon D, et al (1995) Protective effect of fruits and vegetables on development of stroke in men. J Am Med Assoc 273:1113–1117.

61. Key TJ, Thorogood M, Appleby PN, et al (1996) Dietary habits and mortality in 11,000 vegetarians and health conscious people: results of a 17 year follow up. Br Med J 313:775–779.

62. Pietinen P, Rimm EB, Korhonen P, et al (1996) Intake of dietary fiber and risk of coronary heart disease in a cohort of Finnish men. The Alpha-Tocopherol, Beta-Carotene Cancer Prevention Study. Circulation 94:2720–2727.

63. Rimm EB, Ascherio A, Giovannucci E, et al (1996) Vegetable, fruit, and cereal fiber intake and risk of coronary heart disease among men. J Am Med Assoc 275:447–451.

64. Fuchs CS, Stampfer MJ, Coditz GA, et al (1995) Alcohol consumption and mortality among women. N Engl J Med 332:1245–1250.

65. Rimm EB (1996) Alcohol consumption and coronary heart disease: good habits may be more important than just good wine. Am J Epidemiol 143:1094–1097.

66. Rimm EB, Williams P, Fosher K, Criqui M, Stampfer MJ (1999) Moderate alcohol consumption and lower risk of coronary heart disease: meta-analysis of effects on lipids and haemostatic factors. Br Med J 319:1523–1528.

67. Longnecker MP (1994) Alcoholic beverage consumption in relation to risk of breast cancer: meta-analysis and review. Cancer Causes Control 5:73–82.

68. Thun MJ, Peto R, Lopez AD, et al (1997) Alcohol consumption and mortality among middle-aged and elderly U.S. adults. N Engl J Med 337:1705–1714.
69. Willett WC, Stampfer MJ (1997) Sobering data on alcohol and breast cancer. Epidemiology 8:225–227.
70. Hubert HB, Feinleib M, McNamara PM, et al (1983) Obesity as an independent risk factor for cardiovascular disease: a 26-year follow-up of participants in the Framingham Heart Study. Circulation 67: 968–977.
71. Krauss RM, Winston M. (1998) Obesity: impact on cardiovascular disease. Circulation 98:1472–1476.
72. Willett WC, Manson JE, Stampfer MJ, et al (1995) Weight, weight change, and coronary heart disease in women. Risk within the 'normal' weight range. J Am Med Assoc 273:461–465.
73. Nathan DM, Cleary PA, Backlund JY, et al (2005) Intensive diabetes treatment and cardiovascular disease in patients with type 1 diabetes. N Engl J Med 353:2643–2653.
74. UK Prospective Diabetes Study (UKPDS) Group (1998) Intensive blood-glucose control with sulphonylureas or insulin compared with conventional treatment and risk of complications in patients with type 2 diabetes (UKPDS 33). UK Prospective Diabetes Study (UKPDS) Group. Lancet 352:837–853.
75. Berger JS, Roncaglioni MC, Avanzini F, et al (2006) Aspirin for the primary prevention of cardiovascular events in women and men. J Am Med Assoc 295:306–313.
76. US Preventive Services Task Force (2002) Aspirin for the primary prevention of cardiovascular events: recommendations and rationale. Ann Int Med 136:157–160.
77. US Preventive Services Task Force. Guide to Clinical Preventive Services, 3rd ed, 2000–2002. www.ahrq.gov/clinic/prevnew.htm Accessed 11 April 2008.
78. Antithrombotic Trialists' Collaboration (2002) Collaborative meta-analysis of randomized trials of antiplatelet therapy for prevention of death, myocardial infarction and stroke in high-risk patients. Br Med J 324:71–86.
79. Freemantle N, Cleland J, Young P, et al (1999) B blocker after myocardial infarction: systematic review and meta regression analysis. Br Med J 318:1730–1737.
80. Yusuf S, Sleight P, Pogue J, et al (2000) Effects of an angiogenesis-converting-enzyme inhibitor, ramipril, on cardiovascular events in high-risk patients. N Engl J Med 342:145–153.

Chapter 3
Heart Failure in Women

Jaekyoung Hong and Gladys Velarde

INTRODUCTION

Over 5 million Americans are currently affected with heart failure (HF) and well over 50% of these are women. Each year more than 500,000 new cases of HF are diagnosed with and estimated direct and indirect cost over 30 billion dollars. HF has thus emerged as the most serious cardiac problem in the United States. Despite advances in medical management and improved prognosis, HF has high mortality with 37% of men and 33% of women dying within 2 years of diagnosis and a 6-year mortality rate of 82% and 67% for men and women, respectively.[1] Although mortality with heart failure is lower among women than men, women now account for the majority (62.5%) of deaths from HF in the US because of shifting demographics.[2,3]

Despite women accounting for more than one-half of patients with heart failure, they are significantly underrepresented in clinical trials. Subset analyses of large-scale trials have attempted to provide insight into gender related differences in clinical profiles and predictors of outcome, but individually, these analyses are limited by small numbers of female participants, by differing etiologies of HF used, and by the lack of separation of patients with preserved and impaired left ventricular systolic function.

Some of the gender differences in HF can be explained by the trend that women with HF present at an older age and have a lower prevalence of ischemic heart disease and previous myocardial infarction (MI) than men. Women are more likely to have hypertension and be diabetic. Diabetic women have almost double the cardiovascular (CV) mortality than diabetic men and four times the mortality

J.D. Bisognano et al. (eds.), *Manual of Heart Failure Management,*
DOI: 10.1007/978-1-84882-185-9_3, © Springer-Verlag London Limited 2009

than women without diabetes. In addition, women are more likely to develop HF with preserved left ventricular ejection fraction (LVEF) which can be more difficult to diagnose and therefore, more likely to be inadequately treated. These discrepancies may in part explain why women admitted with HF, despite a better survival, have lower health-related quality of life, have more recurrent hospitalizations, and tend to have smaller improvement over their hospitalizations.

This chapter will discuss various causes of HF in women and address challenges with diagnosis, management, and treatment of HF in this population.

CAUSES OF HF IN WOMEN

Hypertension

Hypertension (HTN) is an important risk factor for HF in both men and women.

In multiple large population scale studies examining various risk factors of HF, hypertension has the greatest attributable risk in both men and women for the development of future HF (Figure 3.1). According to the Framingham Study, more women than men had HTN before HF. In this cohort, hypertension preceded the development of HF in 59% of women vs. 39% in men.[5]

Higher prevalence of HTN-induced HF in women is not clearly defined in all studies and it varies depending on numbers of subjects studied, clinical criteria used for diagnosis (LVEF vs. broad symptoms), and self-reported status. Some studies have suggested less optimal blood pressure control for women; however, the National Health and Nutrition Examination Survey (NHANES) data have shown blood pressure control often is better in women than in men.[6] Other studies have theorized that systolic BP with age increases more rapidly in women after menopause and that the prevalence of HTN is higher in women older than 55 years which most likely leads to higher prevalence of HF.

A particular group of women at a higher risk of HF is non-Hispanic black women.

A recent study has shown that for African-American women older than 60 years of age, the group with the highest prevalence of hypertension, the race difference in HF was explained by greater prevalence of HTN and DM in this group of women. However in a younger than 60-year-old women population, African-American race was a predictor of increased risk for HF even after adjusting for DM, HTN, LVH on ECG, and BMI.[6,7]

This finding underscores the complex etiology of HF, especially in this racial group. This in part may be due to socioeconomic

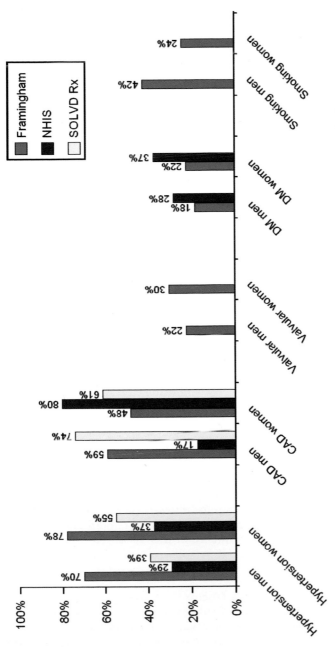

FIGURE 3.1. Prevalence of risk factors in the HF population in the NHIS, Framingham, and SOLVD studies[4].

factors such as low income, limited access to healthcare, sedentary lifestyle, and dietary intake high in salt and saturated fats. Nonetheless, HTN plays an important role in HF in women but especially in younger African-American women.

There appears to be gender differences in the relative contribution of systolic and pulse pressure to the development of HF, with systolic hypertension being more predictive of HF in women and pulse pressure more predictive in men. The relationship of systolic and pulse pressure as risks for heart failure have been more clearly established than that of diastolic pressure. According to the subset of the Framingham study which examined 894 men and 1,146 women with mean age of 61 for new-onset heart failure who were monitored for 18 years, the strongest correlation existed between systolic and pulse pressure with developing HF. For 11.8% of participants who developed HF, a 20 mmHg increment in the systolic pressure correlated to 56% increased risk for HF with hazard ratio of 1.56. Similarly, 16 mmHg or 1 SD pulse pressure conferred 55% increased risk for HF with hazard ratio of 1.55.[8]

Heart failure with normal ejection fraction, frequently termed diastolic HF, is mainly a disease of elderly women, most of whom have hypertension. HF in this group of women is becoming increasingly recognized. Hypertension is indeed the main cause of Heart failure with normal ejection fraction. Prognosis of HF with normal ejection fraction, although better than in systolic dysfunction, is poor. The Framingham Study and the Cardiovascular Health Study revealed annual mortality of 15–19% in systolic HF, 8–9% in HF with normal ejection fraction vs. 1–4% in matched controls without HF.[9]

Gender differences have also been noted in cardiac remodeling during pressure-overload states like severe aortic stenosis (AS). Women with AS tend to develop more cardiac hypertrophy, while men have less hypertrophy, greater ventricular cavity size, and reduced left ventricular function. Histological differences with less degree of fibrosis, apoptosis, and myocyte necrosis has been observed in women with AS compared to men with the same pathology and this may also explain the differences in LV remodeling.[10]

Although hypertension may be a more common cause of HF in women due to a high prevalence of this disease, a woman's individual risk of developing HF is still greater with coronary artery disease (CAD).[4]

Ischemic Coronary Artery Disease

CAD is an important risk factor for HF yet it is less often identified in women because of atypical symptoms and erroneous perceptions. Patients with ischemic cardiomyopathy defined by presence of CAD and LV dysfunction are at increased risk for HF and sudden cardiac death. Systolic HF is more common in women with CAD than those with nonischemic heart disease. The prevalence of CAD in women with HF ranges from 8 to 74% (Figure 3.1) and is less frequent in women than men.[7,11] In the Coronary Artery Surgery Study (CASS) registry, ischemic heart disease HF patients had a worse prognosis than those with nonischemic HF. The prognosis worsened with increased severity of CAD.[11,12] Some studies have suggested that women tend to survive longer than men when HF is due to nonischemic causes, but the mortality in women is comparable with men with ischemic cardiomyopathy.[13] A recent pooled analysis of five randomized control trials suggests that better survival is also seen among women with ischemic cardiomyopathy compared with men in a population with similar ejection fraction with the greatest gender-related survival difference seen between nonischemic women and men.[14] The long-term prognosis appears to be worse for post-myocardial infarction (MI) African-American women who have a higher chance of developing HF and increased mortality within 1 year.[15] In the setting of acute MI, diabetic women are also more likely to develop HF and have a worse prognosis. In general, women are less likely to undergo revascularization than men but if they do, they have higher incidence of HF and mortality after the procedure. They are less likely to receive aspirin, and thrombolytics, although equally likely to receive beta-blockers. Women post-MI, with or without HF, are also less likely to be referred to cardiac rehabilitation. Some of these past inadequacies in the treatment of CAD in older women have contributed to the high prevalence and incidence of HF among older women today.

DM

Diabetes mellitus is a significant risk factor for HF in both genders but more for women, especially younger women. A higher risk ratio for HF for diabetic women compared to diabetic men has been shown in several studies (Figure 3.1).

The Framingham Heart Study was the initial study demonstrating increased risk for CHF in patients with diabetes. In this study, the incidence of HF was 4–5 times higher in diabetic compared to nondiabetic women and that of young diabetic women (age 35–64) was twice as high as in young diabetic men.[16] In addition, multiple studies have shown this association. In a study by Nichols which evaluated the prevalence, incidence, and risk factors for CHF in 9,500 patients with diabetes, HF was prevalent in 11.8% of diabetic patients when compared with 4.5% of nondiabetic patients;

however, the incidence increased significantly with age with HF doubling from 33 cases per 1,000 for 45–54 year-old patient group to 68 cases per 1,000 for 55–64 year-old patient group and 135 cases per 1,000 for 65–74 year-old patient group.[17] The study concluded that HF patients were significantly older, had a longer duration of diabetes (6.4 vs. 4.5 years), were more likely insulin dependent (34.6 yrs vs. 17.7yrs), and were more of women than men (53.8% vs. 47.8%).[4] Also, based on mortality trends in men and women with self-reported diabetes, the CVD mortality rate including HF mortality among diabetic women did not change in the past 25 years unlike that of men with diabetes who showed 43% relative reduction in the age-adjusted mortality rate. The presence of diabetes is also a strong predictor of increased mortality in women with HF and CAD. When HF develops, 25% of diabetic women experience a recurrent MI or a fatal coronary event, more than doubling the rate of nondiabetic women. The reasons for this increased risk are unclear. Several factors can explain why women with diabetes may have a higher mortality rate. These range from inadequate primary prevention of other risk factors, inadequate treatment for CAD when already present, to complex pathophysiologic effects of DM in cardiac muscle. Several studies have cited inadequate therapy with antihypertensive and aspirin therapy and less aggressive revascularization and hospitalization for heart disease in diabetic women with CAD. Also, gender difference in the effect of DM in LV mass, wall stress, arterial stiffness, and autonomic dysfunction as well as differences in the coronary microvasculature, endothelial dysfunction, metabolic affect on myocytes, and in inflammatory and hormonal responses to DM likely play an important role.[18] Given that women are more likely to develop HF with preserved LV ejection fraction, a lack of recognition and therefore treatment of HF may also play a role in their higher mortality.

Valvular Heart Disease

Valvular heart disease accounts roughly for about 8% of HF cases. For women it appears that this number is slightly lower at about 5% but accurate data is sparse.[19] There is a gender influence in the prevalence of some types of valvular heart disease.[20] For example, rheumatic mitral stenosis due to rheumatic fever in childhood used to be a major cause of valve disease in women. This still is a major contributor of HF in some part of the underdeveloped world. In developed countries, a more common cause of HF is due to degenerative valvular disease with AS being the classic example. Mitral valve prolapse (MVP), which affects roughly 6% of all women, is the most common form of valve disease in women. Often times,

MVP does not progress to HF and therefore will not require treatment. Mitral stenosis (MS) can be caused by rheumatic fever, infectious endocarditis, SLE, and degenerative myxomatous changes. MS can present with HF symptoms especially in the young where the stenosis becomes unmasked by higher hemodynamic demands under certain physiologic conditions like pregnancy, thyrotoxicosis, or severe anemia. According to Redberg et al., Women account for almost 70% of patients with diagnoses of aortic or mitral valve disease.[21] In addition, more than 60% of heart valve replacement procedures are performed in women.[21] Degenerative AS unlike MS is a disease of elderly patients and affects men and women equally. In degenerative AS, several physiopathological differences have been reported in women: the amount of calcium is lower than in men and the left ventricle generates higher gradients and hypercontractile response in women. Valve disease such as high grade MS or AS can pose a risk for women (and fetus) in pregnancy mainly because of the increased cardiac output during pregnancy and during labor, increased plasma volume which results in anemia, and increased heart rate which decreases filling time. The hemodynamic changes of pregnancy in women with preexisting cardiac lesions can result in serious complications including mortality. The New York Heart Association functional classification is used as a predictor of outcome. Women with NYHA class III and IV face a mortality rate of 7% and morbidity over 30%.[22] Additionally, HF as indicated by NYHA functional class greater than II and/or LV dysfunction of EF <40% were risk factors highly predictive of adverse cardiac or neonatal complications in a study of about 300 women with heart disease.[23]

It has also been seen consistently in the literature that women undergoing cardiac surgery in general, coronary or valvular, have higher mortality rates than men especially in the early postoperative period. The reasons for this increased mortality are not entirely clear.

Peripartum Cardiomypathy
Peripartum cardiomypathy (PPCM) is a unique condition which occurs in 1 in 3,000–4,000 births. PPCM is defined by reduced LVEF in women within last month of pregnancy and/or up to the first 5 months of postpartum.[24] These women do not have any prior cardiac history and may present with fatigue, dyspnea on exertion, and edema. For 50–60% of women, they completely recover normal heart size and function within 6 months of delivery.[25] However, LV dysfunction can persist and it can also deteriorate. Digoxin, diuretics, and hydralazine can be used during

pregnancy and while breastfeeding. B-blockers are considered to be safe, but there have been case reports of growth retardation and fetal bradycardia associated with them so they should be used with caution. Anticoagulation can be considered in patients with severe cardiomyopathy, but ACE inhibitors are contraindicated. Women with persistent PPCM who have subsequent pregnancy have higher risk of maternal morbidity and mortality. Risk factors for PPCM include: advanced maternal age, multiparity, multifetal pregnancy, African-American race, preeclampsia, and gestational hypertension.[25] Patients with PPCM who fail medical therapy may be candidates for heart transplantation.

Chemotherapy

Cardiotoxicity due to cytotoxic drugs can cause severe morbidity and mortality in cancer patients. Formation of free oxygen radials and disturbed mitochondrial energy metabolism are thought to be key factors in the pathogenesis of the cardiotoxicity, of anthracycline-based regimens. Anthracycline chemotherapy is commonly used for the treatment of breast, uterine, and ovarian cancers and thus present unique challenges to cancer treatment in women.[26] The risk of HF in women treated with anthracycline-based regimens, primarily for breast cancer, has increased and unfortunately remains large underestimated. The anthracycline-induced cardiomyopathy is a common adverse effect of the medication and can cause dose-dependent impairment of LV function. With the upper limit of 550 mg/m2 cumulative dose, early HF may develop in 30% of the patients receiving the high dosages.[26] The onset of the cardiotoxicity can range from immediately after the treatment to several years after the therapy. Therefore, a close follow up is required to monitor the onset of the disease. Although the anthracycline-induced heart failure is considered to be irreversible, more studies have shown that HF medical therapy may have some benefit on improvement of heart failure.[27] The cardiotoxicity of these drugs is a serious side effect and the treatment/management of HF in these patients require further studies.

Depression

Depression is frequently associated with heart failure and is more common in elderly women.[28,29] The higher prevalence of HF may be due to medical noncompliance or difficulty distinguishing between symptoms of ischemic heart disease and depression such as dyspnea, fatigue, anorexia, chest discomfort, or palpitation. With acute stress, transient changes in blood pressure has been established, but is unclear why type of hemodynamic changes or sympathetic overdrive may be linked to depression-induced HF. In a recent 14 year follow-up-study which screened for HF in patients with depression, Williams and colleagues showed that depression can be a cause of heart failure,[28] After excluding a little more than 300 patients who met the study's definition of preexisting heart failure, the study population comprised of approximately 1,000 men and nearly 1,500 women whose average age was 74. Controlling for cofounders such as CAD, DM, and HTN, the study showed that about 20% of the depressed women developed HF compared with 10% of the nondepressed women. In comparison, only 12% depressed men developed HF compared to 15% of the nondepressed men.[28] The association between depression and HF is not clear and requires further investigation.

SYMPTOMS AND DIAGNOSIS OF HF IN WOMEN

Common symptoms of HF are fatigue, dyspnea, orthopnea, paroxysmal nocturnal dyspnea (PND), and exercise intolerance as shown on Table 3.1.

On physical exam, crackles, nonproductive cough, and S3/4 gallops may be found, but the sensitivity and the specificity of these physical exam findings may not be reliable.

(Table 3.1). The signs or symptoms are the same in women and men, but women are more likely to have dyspnea, edema, elevated jugular venous pressure, and an audible S3 gallop.[30]

TABLE 3.1. Table showing the sensitivity and specificity of signs and physical exam findings of heart failure (adapted from the Field Guide to Bedside Diagnosis, Copyright © 2007 Lippincott Williams & Wilkins)

Sign	Sensitivity	Specificity	Likelihood
Increased left ventricular filling pressure			
Abnormal valsalva response	95	88	7.6
Third heart sounds (S_3)	12–32	95–96	5.7
Abdominojugular reflux	87	83	5.1
JVD	59	86	4.2
Rales	64	84	4.0
Edema	10	93	1.4
Decreased left ventricular10 ejection fraction			
Abnormal valsalva response	69–88	90–91	7.6
Third heart sounds (S_3)	14	96	7.0
Displaced apex	39	93	5.6
Orthopnea	97	64	2.7
DOE NYHA 3–4	42	84–89	2.6
Rales	14	93	2.0

It is difficult to distinguish systolic and diastolic HF based on symptoms and signs of HF alone. Measurement of neurohormonal levels such as B-type natriuretic peptide (BNP) may aid in the diagnosis of HF, but women tend to have a higher "normal value" than men.[31] Diastolic heart failure describes a clinical syndrome whereas diastolic dysfunction describes a mechanical abnormality of the LV. Diastolic dysfunction is a consequence of longstanding and poorly controlled hypertension and it is characterized by concentric remodeling with preserved LV end diastolic volume, increased passive ventricular stiffness, and abnormalities of active relaxation(Table 3.2).[32]

Because of the difficulty measuring diastolic function and lack of clear diagnostic criteria for diastolic heart failure, the term heart failure with preserved left ventricular systolic function is used and is often preferred. Despite greater prevalence of systolic HF in men, women and elderly patients (often overlapping populations) are more likely to have HF with preserved LV systolic function. Among elderly women population, more than 50% of the patients have HF with preserved EF.[32]

The diagnosis of diastolic dysfunction is made based on symptoms and signs of HF with normal LV ejection fraction and no valvular dysfunction on echocardiography.

MANAGEMENT OF HF IN WOMEN

Current recommendations for HF therapy are not gender-specific given the lack of large randomized gender-specific blinded studies. Similarly the treatment for patients with HF and preserved LV systolic function remains limited and often requires therapy for the underlying cause. Current guidelines are therefore based on patients with systolic HF and thus should be interpreted with caution when applying them to those with preserved LV systolic function. The role of ACEI, ARBs, statins, antiplatelet therapy, and beta-blockers are well established by multiple trials in patients with LV dysfunction. Although gender differences in survival with ACE inhibitor therapy have been reported, the small numbers of women and lack of direct comparison with men have limited this observation. Similarly concerns about digoxin arose after post hoc analyses of the DIG trial showed a trend toward worse outcome in women on this therapy.[33]

For the management of HF with preserved systolic function, there are only a few studies with ACE inhibitors, ARBs, digitalis, diuretics, beta-blockers, and calcium channel blockers. Most of the studies are small and inconclusive. The only large-scale randomized clinical trial comparing a drug therapy to placebo in patients with

TABLE 3.2. Characteristics of systolic HF compared to diastolic HF[32]

Characteristics	Diastolic HF	Systolic HF
Age	Predominantly in the elderly	Any age, mainly 50–70 yrs
Gender	Predominantly in women	Predominantly in men
Gallop rhythm	S_4	S_3
LV EF	>45%	=45%
LV diameter	Usually NL or LVH	Usually dilated
ECG – LVH	Common	Common
ECG – LBBB, grade III	Uncommon	Common
ECG – Old MI	Uncommon	Common
ECG – Atrial fibrillation	Paroxysmal/Persistent	Persistent
CXR	Congestion with or without cardiomegaly	Congestion and cardiomegaly
Preexistent conditions		
Arterial hypertension	+++	++
DM	+++	++
Previous MI	+	+++
Obesity	+++	+
Chronic pulmonary disease	++	0
Chronic dialysis	++	0
In-hospital mortality	3–5%	5–10%
Rehospitalizations	50% in 1 year	50% in 1 year
Presentation forms		
Acute HF	Hypertensive acute edema, occasionally acute MI	Acute MI, valvulopathies and myocarditis
Decompensated chronic HF	Hypertensive acute edema	Congestive syndromes

0 Absent, + Little frequent, ++ Frequent, +++ Very frequent.

diastolic HF is the CHARM-PRESERVED trial. Compared to the patients with low EF in the two trials of CHARM, in CHARM-PRESERVED there was a higher proportion of women (40%), higher prevalence of HTN and less likely to report a previous MI. The study showed that while Candesartan may help in preventing admissions for congestive HF, the CV mortality did not decrease during the 36 month mean follow up in patients with HF and LVEF > 40%. Other studies, such as the irbesartan in heart failure with preserved systolic function (I-PRESERVE) and the treatment of preserved cardiac function HF with an aldosterone antagonist (TOPCAT), may shed new light into the medical therapy of this difficult to manage patient population, most of which is women and elderly. Currently, the management of diastolic HF focuses on symptoms and underlying causes of HF such as HTN, Diabetes, and/or ischemia. Maintenance of sinus rhythm or rate control in patient with atrial fibrillation may also play an important role.

Another line of therapy is implantable cardioverter defibrillators (ICDs). This therapy is recommended for primary prevention of sudden cardiac death in patients with mild to moderate HF symptoms and left ventricular ejection fraction of less than 30–35%.

In the MADIT-II trial, ICD therapy was better than medical therapy in survival outcome of patients with ischemic HF. The majority of the patients (86%) in the MADIT-II trial were men. In the analysis of the MADIT-II trial which examined the cardiac events in post-MI patients with ICD therapy, it was shown that women were more likely to have comorbidities such as HTN and DM and less likely to have had coronary artery bypass grafting. The mortality within 2 years was not different between men and women, but the risk of ICD therapy such as arrhythmic events were lower in women.

The ICD therapy has been recognized as life saving and in 2004, the Medicare criteria for coverage of ICD for primary prevention was expanded to cover patients with NYHA class II or III HF and LVEF <30%.[34] Yet, according to Hernandez and colleagues, women and racial/ethnic minorities were less likely to have an ICD implanted. Compared to Caucasian men, African-American men were 73% likely to have an ICD.[35] For Caucasian women and African-American women with ischemic HF, the percentages were 62% and 56%, respectively.[35] Given the small number of women and minorities in studies, the question of whether the lower ICD implantation rates in women and minorities lead to worse outcomes remains unanswered. Although, for older patients, there are concerns that ICD therapy may not provide the mortality benefit.

A recent analysis of ICD implants in Canada showed patients aged 65–74 years receiving ICDs may have increased risk of mortality and those 75 years or older may possibly have threefold increase in risk of death compared to 65 years old patients.[36]

Cardiac resynchronization therapy (CRT) or biventricular pacing is another therapy that has been shown in some large prospective randomized multicenter trials to improve HF symptoms, LV ejection fraction, and mortality rates. Although very few studies have reported gender-specific data, the technique appears to be beneficial for both men and women.

CONCLUSIONS

The diagnosis and treatment of HF in women remains challenging. Women are more likely to be older, diabetic, and hypertensive. Women are also more likely to have nonischemic HF, have preserved systolic function, and are more likely to have more symptoms. Because of the high mortality associated with HF in both women and men, identifying and treating modifiable risk factors such as HTN, DM, and CAD early is an important strategy in prevention of HF. The difficulty in diagnosis of HF with preserved systolic function along with less established treatment options highlights the need for more large-scale trials in diagnosing and managing this particular population.

References

1. Rosamond W, Flegal K, Friday G, Furie K, Go A, Greenlund K, Haase N, Ho M, Howard V, Kissela B, Kittner S, Lloyd-Jones D, McDermott M, Meigs J, Moy C, Nichol G, O'Donnell CJ, Roger V, Rumsfeld J, Sorlie P, Steinberger J, Thom T, Wasserthiel-Smoller S, Hong Y. Heart disease and stroke statistics: 2007 update: a report from the American Heart Association Statistics Committee and Stroke Statistics Subcommittee. *Circulation* 2007;115:e172.
2. American Heart Association. Heart Disease and Stroke Statistics 2006 Update. Dallas, TX: American Heart Association, 2005.
3. Levy D, Kenshaiah S, Larson M. Long term trends in the incidence of and survival with heart failure. *N Engl J Med* 2002;347:1397–1402.
4. Lund LH, Mancini D. Hear failure in women. *Med Clin North Am* 2004;88:1321–1345.
5. Levy D, Larson MG, Vasan RS, Kannel WB, Ho KK. The progression from hypertension to congestive heart failure. *J Am Med Assoc* 1996; 275:1557–1562.
6. Franklin S, Jacobs M, Wong N, L'Italien G, Laperta P. Predominance of isolated systolic hypertension among middle-aged and elderly US hypertensives. *Hypertension* 2001;37:869–874.
7. Richard G. Epidemiology of hypertension in African American women: Progress in cardiology. *Am Heart J* 131(2):385–395.

8. Haider AW, Larson MG, Franklin SS, Levy D. Systolic blood pressure, diastolic blood pressure, and pulse pressure as predictors of risk for congestive heart failure in the Framingham Heart Study. *Ann Intern Med* 2003;138:10–16.

9. Vasan Rs, Larson MG, Benjamin EJ, Evans JC, Reiss CK, Levy D. Congestive heart failure in subjects with normal versus reduced left ventricular ejection fraction: prevalence and mortality in a population-based cohort. *J Am Coll Cardiol* 1999;33:1948–1955.

10. Guerra S, Leri A, Wang X, et al. Myocyte death in the failing human heart is gender dependent. *Cir Res.* 1999;85:856–866.

11. Johnstone D, Limacher M, Liang C, Ekelund L. Clinical characteristics of patients in Studies of Left Ventricular Dysfunction (SOLVD). *Am J Cardiol* 1992;70:894–900.

12. Redfield M, Jacobsen S, Burnett J, Mahoney D, Bailey K, Rodeheffer R. Buren of systolic and diastolic ventricular dysfunction in the community. *J Am Med Assoc* 2003;289:194–202.

13. Sweitzer N, Loptain M, Yancy C, Mills R, Stevenson L. Comparison of clinical features and outcomes of patients hospitalized with heart failure and normal ejection fraction versus those with mildly reduced and moderately to severely reduced fractions. *Am J Cardiol* 2008;101:1151–1156.

14. Frazier CG, Alexander KP, Newby K, Anderson S, Iverson E, Packer M, Cohn J, Goldstein S, Douglas PS. Associations of gender and etiology with outcomes in heart failure with systolic dysfunction. A pooled analysis of 5 randomized control trials. *J Am Coll Cardiol* 2007;49:1450–1458.

15. Lund A, Mancini D. Heart failure in women. *Med Clin N Am* 2004; 1321–1345.

16. Kannel WB, Hjortland M, Castelli WP. Role of diabetes in congestive heart failure: the Framingham study. *Am J Cardiol* 1974;34:29–34.

17. Nichols G, Hillier T, Erbey J, Brown J. Congestive heart failure in type 2 diabetes: prevalence, incidence and risk factors. *Diabetes Care* 2001;24:1614–1619.

18. Bonow RO, Mitch WE, Nesto RW, O'Gara PT, Becker RC, Clark LT, Hunt S, Jialal I, Lipshultz SE, Loh E. Prevention Conference VI: Diabetes and Cardiovascular Disease: Writing Group V: management of cardiovascular-renal complications. *Circulation* 2002;105:e159–e164.

19. Tornos P. Valvular heart disease in women. *Rev Esp Cardiol* 2006;59: 832–836.

20. Bonow RO, Carabello BA, deLeon AC, et al. ACC/AHA guidelines for the management of patients with valvular heart disease: a report of the American College of Cardiology/American Heart Association Task Force on Practice Guidelines (Committee on management of patients with valvular heart disease). *J Am Coll Cardiol* 1998;32:1486–1588.

21. Redberg R, Schiller N. Gender and valvular surgery. *J Thorac Cardiovasc Surg* 2004;127:1–3.

22. Stout K, Otto C. Pregnancy in women with valvular heart disease. *Heart* 2007;93:552–558.

23. Siu SC, Colman JM, Sorensen S, Smallhorn JF, Farine D, Amankwah KS, Spears JC, Sermer M. Adverse neonatal and cardiac outcomes are more common in pregnant women with cardiac disease. *Circulation* 2002;105:2170–2184

24. Veille J. Peripartum cardiomyopathies: a review. *Am J Obstet Gynecol* 1984; 148:805–818.

25. Demakis JG, Rahimtoola SH, Sutton GC, Meadows WR, Szanto PB, Tobin JR, Gunnar RM. Natural course of peripartum cardiomyopathy. *Circulation* 1971;44:1053–1061.

26. Rhoden W, Hasleton P, Brooks N, Anthracyclines and the heart. *Br Heart J* 1993;70:499–502.

27. Saini J, Rich MW, and Lyss AP, Reversibility of severe left ventricular dysfunction due to doxorubicin cardiotoxicity. Report of three cases. *Ann Intern Med* 1987;106:814–816.

28. Williams SA, Kasl SV, Heiat A, Abramson JL, Krumholz HM, Vaccarino V. Depression and risk of heart failure among the elderly: a prospective Community-based study. *Psychosom Med* 2002;64:6–12.

29. Mendes de Leon CF, Krumholz HM, Seeman TS, Vaccarino V, Williams CS, Kasl SV. Depression and risk of coronary heart disease in elderly men and women. *Arch Intern Med* 1998; 158: 2341–2348.

30. Johnstone D, Limacher M, Rousseau M, . Clinical characteristics of patients in studies of left ventricular dysfunction (SOLVD). *Am J Cardiol* 1992:70:894–900.

31. Redfield MM, Rodeheffer RJ, Jacobsen SJ, Mahoney DW, et al. Plasma brain natriuretic peptide concentration:impact of age and gender. *J Am Coll Cardiol* 2002:40:976–982.

32. Goldstein SR, Dick C. Differentiating systolic from diastolic heart failure: pathophysiology and therapeutic considerations. *Am J Med* 1993;95:645–655.

33. Rathore SS, Wang Y, Krumholz HM. Sex-based differences in the effect of digocin for the treatment of heart failure. *N Engl J Med* 2002:347:1403–1411.

34. Al-Khatib SM. Does ICD therapy benefit women with a history of myocardial infarction and severe left ventricular dysfunction? *J Cardiovasc Electrophysiol* 2005;16:1271–1272.

35. Hernandez AF, Fonarow GC, Liang L, Al-Khatib SM, Curtis LH, LaBresh KA, Yancy CW, Albert NA, Peterson ED. Sex and racial differences in the implantable cardioverter defibrillators among patients hospitalized with heart failure. *J Am Med Assoc* 2007;298:1525–1532.

36. Healey JS, Hallstrom AP, Karl-Heinz K, Nair S, Schron EP, Roberts RS, Morillo CA, Connolly SJ. Role of the implantable defibrillator among elderly patients with a history of life-threatening ventricular arrhythmias. *Eur Heart J* 2007;28:1746–1749.

Chapter 4
Systolic Heart Failure

J. Chad Teeters and Jeffrey D. Alexis

In the most basic terms, systolic heart failure is the inability of the heart to supply the body's tissues with enough blood to meet metabolic demands. This process has been recognized for centuries, and one of the first descriptions dates back to the twelfth century in a biography of the Byzantine emperor Alexius I Comnenus that detailed his symptoms as follows:

> *Every day it grew worse, attacking him no longer at intervals, but relentlessly, with no interruption. He was unable to lie on either side, so weak that every breath involved great effort... his condition was serious, for never for one moment could he breathe freely. He was forced to sit upright in order to breathe at all; if by chance he did lie on his back or side, the suffocation was awful: to breathe in or exhale even a tiny stream of air became impossible.*[1]

Although the understanding and treatment of this disease has come quite a long way since this report, the untreated symptoms and effect they have upon patients suffering with this process remain unchanged.

It is estimated that heart failure afflicts approximately 5 million people in the United States currently with an additional 550,000 incident cases each year.[2] Further, it is a disease that demonstrates a predilection for the elderly with an estimated 10 out of every 1,000 patients over the age of 65.[2] From a societal point of view, there are an estimated 3.6 million admissions for heart failure in the US each year[3] at an estimated cost of 500 million dollars annually.[4] Unfortunately, despite recent therapeutic advances, the five-year mortality of systolic failure remains approximately 60% in men and 45% in women.[5]

J.D. Bisognano et al. (eds.). *Manual of Heart Failure Management,*
DOI: 10.1007/978-1-84882-185-9_4, © Springer-Verlag London Limited 2009

ETIOLOGY

Heart failure is not truly one diagnosis but an endpoint of several etiologic factors. Broadly, there are two etiologies for systolic dysfunction: ischemic cardiomyopathy and non-ischemic cardiomyopathy. Ischemic cardiomyopathy is secondary to coronary artery obstruction with or without myocardial damage leading to reduced cardiac function. Non-ischemic cardiomyopathy has many more possible etiologies (see Table 4.1). Although the pathophysiology of causing systolic dysfunction may differ between the two, treatment of each remains generally the same and both ischemic and non-ischemic cardiomyopathy are associated with significant morbidity and mortality (Table 4.1).

PATHOPHYSIOLOGY

Mechanically, systolic heart failure is due to decreased myocardial contractility leading to higher end-diastolic volumes and pressures, which gradually leads to increased myocardial wall stress resulting in eccentric remodeling. As the heart outwardly remodels, there is a resultant decrease in cross-linking of actin and myosin leading to a net decrease in contractile segments. This phenomenon can perhaps best be understood in relation to the Starling curve (see Figure 4.1). The pressure volume relationships within a normal left ventricle are demonstrated by this relationship. However, in systolic failure, the curve is shifted to the right for the reasons noted above, and visually represented in Figure 4.2.

The reasons for this eccentric remodeling are multifactorial. Despite the etiology, there is always an incipient event leading to the change in ventricular geometry and performance. The initial

TABLE 4.1. Heart failure etiologies

Ischemic	Non-Ischemic
Atherosclerosis	Viral
Diabetes	Tachycardia mediated
Vasospasm	Hypertensive
Arterial inflammation	Valvular
	Post-partum
	Drug-induced
	Hypertensive
	Congenital
	Severe anemia
	Hyperthyroidism
	Hypothyroidism
	Idiopathic

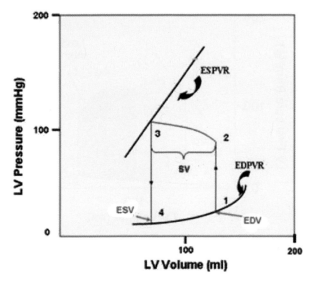

FIGURE 4.1. Starling curve for normal left ventricle (LV). This shows the cardiac cycle phases of ventricular filling (4→1), isovolumetric contraction (1→2), systolic ejection (23) and isovolumetric relaxation (3→4). The end-diastolic volume (EDV) is the maximal volume achieved at the end of filling, and end-systolic volume (ESV) is the minimal volume (i.e., residual volume) of the ventricle found at the end of ejection. The width of the loop, therefore, represents the difference between EDV and ESV, which is defined as the stroke volume (SV). The filling phase moves along the end-diastolic pressure-volume relationship (EDPVR), or passive filling curve for the ventricle. The slope of the EDPVR is the reciprocal of ventricular compliance. The maximal pressure that can be developed by the ventricle at any given left ventricular volume is the end-systolic pressure-volume relationship (ESPVR), which represents the inotropic state of the ventricle.

response to this change is an increase in norepinephrine (NE) to augment myocardial contractility and stimulate the renin-angiotension-aldosterone system (RAAS), which helps to maintain systemic arterial pressure.[7] The myocardium responds to the increase in afterload (i.e., higher systemic pressure) by increasing cyclic-AMP (c-AMP) levels, which increases influx of calcium into the cells. This increase in cytosolic calcium leads to increased contractility and decreased myocardial relaxation.[8] This response is maladaptive and begins a continuous downward spiral in cardiac function and propagates systolic failure. The stimulation of the RAAS system has the secondary effect of increasing salt and

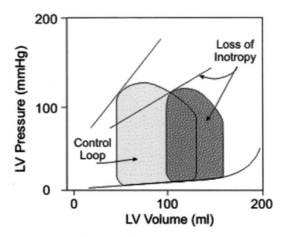

FIGURE 4.2. Normal and systolic failure volume loops. The control loop represents the normal left ventricular pressure-volume loop with a shift to the right along the end-diastolic pressure volume relationship curve for the Loss of Inotropy loop (representing systolic failure). Notice the curve not only showing higher diastolic volumes, but also a smaller stroke volume when compared with the control loop. (Adapted from Klabunde's Cardiovascular Physiology Concepts[6]).

water retention, which increases ventricular preload, and, thus, increases diastolic volume as seen in the pressure volume loops in Figure 4.2. All of these responses lead to increased myocardial energy consumption. As this progresses, the counter-regulatory cytokines (nitric oxide, bradykinin, prostaglandins, atrial natriuretic peptide, and brain natriuretic peptide) become less effective and the effects of the RAAS system go unchecked.[8] The loss of these compensatory mechanisms leads to a state in which the system is unable to respond to acute stresses, and thus minimal stresses can precipitate acute decompensation.

PATIENT PRESENTATION
Similar to the symptoms of Alexius I Comnenus in the twelfth century, patients typically complain of a common clustering of symptoms. These symptoms include progressive weight gain/fluid retention, dyspnea, progressive fatigue, inability to lie flat (orthopnea), and paroxysmal nocturnal dyspnea (PND). Although many patients may present with all of the above, there is no required clustering of symptoms to make the diagnosis of heart failure. As the onset of these symptoms may occur slowly, many patients may

be unaware of some of the above findings. Despite these apparent differences in presentation, what does appear consistent between patients is that as the dysfunction progresses, the degree of exertion required to manifest the symptoms decreases.

EXAM FINDINGS

As there is no reliable clustering of symptoms upon which to base a diagnosis, the physical exam findings are key to making diagnosis of heart failure. Although many patients with stable heart failure may appear quite normal, there may be some subtle findings apparent. Commonly, patients with heart failure will have notable dyspnea secondary to ambulating into the examination room. With more progressive disease or with acute decompensation, patients will appear dyspneic at rest without any preceding exertion. Likewise, one ominous finding in patients with advanced disease is cachexia as wasting with heart failure portends a poor prognosis with a 3-month mortality approaching 20%, and a nearly 40% mortality at 12 months.[8] Cardiac cachexia is defined as a nonvoluntary, non-edematous weight loss of more than 6% over a 6-month period and is found in over 15% of patients with heart failure.[9]

On cardiac examination, there are several more potential clues to the diagnosis. The first is an elevated jugular venous pressure. This may be accentuated during inspiration with increased venous return leading to greater distention of the jugular vein. Next, there may be a compensatory tachycardia present to accommodate for the diminished stroke volume. Systolic blood pressure may be reduced, while the diastolic pressure may be elevated due to poor cardiac output and high resting adrenergic tone, respectively. Finally, there may be an S3 heart sound, best heard at the apex and in the left lateral decubitus position. With more advanced eccentric dilatation, the PMI may also be laterally displaced and diminished due to an enlarged ventricle with less vigorous contraction.

The lung exam is one of the most important components to make a clinical diagnosis of heart failure. The hallmark findings are rales over the lower lung fields, possibly coupled with expiratory wheezing and frothy, blood-tinged sputum expectoration. With more advanced disease or acute decompensation, there may be diminished lung sounds at the bases due to pleural effusions.

Exam of the abdomen may also reveal several findings. First, hepatomegaly may be present due to passive congestion of the liver. Next, compression of the liver may cause increased jugular venous distention (termed hepatojugular reflux). Ascites may also be present, but this is neither required nor specific for the diagnosis of heart failure.

Finally, on examination of the extremities one often finds edema present. This is significant in that most adults will not manifest signs of edema until they experience a gain of at least 5 L of extracellular fluid.[8] Importantly, edema in the absence of rales on pulmonary exam may be more indicative of right ventricular failure, nephritic syndrome, venous insufficiency, or other hypo-oncotic pressure states.

LABORATORY EVALUATION

As the diagnosis of heart failure is purely clinical, there are no imaging modalities or serum studies required to make the diagnosis. Nevertheless, there are important studies that should be monitored in patients with heart failure, and which may add additional information for further management. In mild disease, there is unlikely to be any significant alterations seen in baseline laboratory values. However, with more advanced disease or with medically managed disease, more abnormalities may be seen.

First, in basic serum chemistry studies, one may find elevated BUN and creatinine reflecting renal hypoperfusion due to poor cardiac output. In patients on chronic loop diuretics, one may expect to see hyponatremia reflecting sodium wasting coupled with an inability to excrete water leading to a dilutional state. Similarly, chronic diuretics may result in hypokalemia due to wasting. However, in patients on potassium-sparing diuretics or angiotensin-converting enzyme inhibitors (ACE inhibitors), hyperkalemia may be found.

Liver function studies may reveal elevated aspartate aminotransferase (AST) and alanine aminotransferase (ALT) secondary to hepatic distention. Generalized hyperbilirubinemia may also be seen due to hepatic congestion. In acute decompensation, frank jaundice may also be seen. In chronic failure, elevation of the prothrombin time may reflect impaired hepatic synthesis due to sustained congestion.

Another serum marker of interest is brain natriuretic peptide (BNP). BNP is a 23 amino acid structure, whose main storage site, contrary to what the name implies, is the cardiac ventricles. With an increase in ventricular volume and pressure overload, there is greater release of this substance. Numerous studies have shown a direct correlation between BNP levels and ventricular failure. In fact, levels of over 100 pg/mL have more than a 95% specificity and 98% sensitivity for the diagnosis of heart failure.[8] More recent literature fails to demonstrate a correlation between degree of elevation of BNP and severity of heart failure.

IMAGING STUDIES

Although cardiac imaging can be of utility in making the diagnosis of systolic failure, and certainly may be of benefit in generating a prognosis by determining extent of dysfunction, the most commonly utilized tool is a chest X-ray. PA projection chest radiography is very useful in determining the size of the left ventricle as well as the presence of pulmonary edema (usually noted by cephalization of pulmonary vessels, known as Kerley A lines, and Kerley B lines, see Figure 4.3).

Chest radiography can also give information about the size of the right ventricle as well, as on a lateral projection of the chest, obliteration of the retrosternal air space due to cardiac opacity suggests right ventricular enlargement. Thus, the chest radiograph

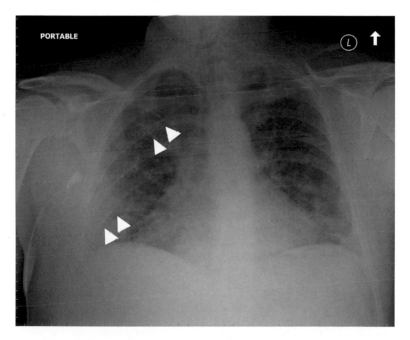

FIGURE 4.3. Chest radiogram in patient with heart failure. In the radiograph above, Kerley A lines (*white arrowheads*) can be seen in the upper lobes of the lung. These *lines* represent engorgement of vessels in the lung apices in response to hypoventilation of the lower lobes due to pulmonary edema and preferential shunting of blood flow toward areas of improved ventilation. Kerley B lines are also seen in the lower lobes (*white arrowheads*) and represent fluid accumulation in the interlobular septae at the lung periphery.

is both relatively inexpensive, and provides significant information that can confirm the clinical diagnosis of heart failure.

Another major imaging modality utilized for diagnosis, management, and prognostication of systolic heart failure is the transthoracic echocardiogram (TTE). The TTE allows for quantification of chamber size (systolic and diastolic), assessment of valvular function, and estimation of left ventricular ejection fraction. This tool can also present clues as to the etiology of systolic dysfunction, and thus aid in the diagnostic work-up.

The electrocardiogram has limited value in heart failure diagnosis or management. It can give clues as to chamber size and hypertrophy as well as conduction delay, which may suggest ventricular dyssynchrony (the management of which will be addressed later in this text, see Chap. 9). In general, it is neither sensitive nor specific for the diagnosis of heart failure, but may be of utility for determining the etiology of systolic dysfunction.

Perhaps the gold standard for evaluation of right and left heart function is right and left heart catheterization. This imaging modality can give real-time estimates of chamber pressures and response to therapy. These results can be followed over time as a marker of both disease progression and therapeutic success. Unfortunately, this imaging modality is invasive and carries a small but definable risk of complications from the procedure, so despite its utility, it is often used sparingly if at all in the diagnosis and management of this disease.

Once the diagnosis of heart failure has been made, there are several staging scales used to assess functional classification. The two most commonly used are the New York Heart Association (NYHA) class scale (see Table 4.2) and the American College of Cardiology and American Heart Association (ACC/AHA) working group staging system (see Table 4.3). These classification systems are similar in that they stratify a patient based upon their functional capabilities with greater disutility being staged higher. The difference between the two is that the NYHA scale is fluctuant and

TABLE 4.2. NYHA heart failure classification scale

Class	Associated symptoms
I	No limitation with ordinary activities
II	Mild limitation of activity; patient is comfortable at rest and with mild exertion
III	Marked limitation of activity; the patient is comfortable only at rest
IV	Any activity brings on dyspnea; symptoms occur at rest

TABLE 4.3. ACC/AHA Heart failure staging system

Stage	Associated events
A	Risk factors for heart failure are present but there are no structural cardiac abnormalities
B	Structural cardiac changes are present but patient is asymptomatic
C	Previous or current symptoms of heart failure with evidence of structural abnormality, but is able to be managed medically
D	Advanced disease requiring hospital-based support; consideration of either transplantation or palliative care is appropriate

patients may move from one level to another with decompensation or therapeutic response. In contrast, the ACC/AHA staging system reflects the worst clustering of symptoms the patient has experienced, and is therefore less fluctuant.

Many other classification systems exist; however, these two are the most commonly cited and used in practice. Management strategies based upon heart failure classification/stage will be discussed later in this text.

References

1. Lutz, JE. A XII century description of congestive heart failure. Am J Cardiol. 61, 494–495 (1988).
2. Heart and Stroke Statistical Update, American Heart Association (2002).
3. U.S. Heart Failure Program is Saving Lives, U.S. Department of Health and Human Services (2007).
4. Lenz TL, Hilleman DE. Nesiritide usage in decompensated heart failure: Cost effectiveness and clinical effectiveness. Heart Drug. 5:81–88 (2005)
5. Chiang WK, Talavera F, Setnik G, Halamka J, Brenner B. Congestive Heart Failure and Pulmonary Edema. http://www.emedicine.com/emerg/TOPIC108.HTM, May, 2006.
6. Klabunde, RE. Cardiovascular Physiology Concepts. http://www.cvphysiology.com/Heart%20Failure/HF005.htm (2007)
7. Zevitz, ME. Heart Failure. eMedicine, http://www.emedicine.com/MED/topic3552.htm. (2006).
8. Anker SD, Ponikowski P, Varney S, et al. Wasting as independent risk factor of survival in chronic heart failure. Lancet. 349:1050–1053 (1997).
9. Springer J, Filippatos G, Akashi YJ, Anker SD. Prognosis and therapy approaches of cardiac cachexia. Curr Opin Cardiol. 21(3):229–33 (2006)

Chapter 5
Heart Failure with Preserved Ejection Fraction

James Gallagher and Michael Fong

INTRODUCTION

In 2007, it was estimated that the United States would spend $33.2 billion dollars on both the direct and indirect costs of heart failure (HF). In 2004, hospital discharges for HF numbered 1,099,000 up from 399,000, twenty-five years prior. In 2002, total-mention mortality for HF was 296,700 people.[1] The proportion of patients with heart failure with preserved ejection fraction (HFPEF) is increasing over time, and unlike those with reduced systolic function, survival is not appreciably improving.[2] In addition, despite the growing prevalence, few well-designed, large clinical trials exist.[3,4] This chapter is intended to define heart failure in the setting of preserved ejection fraction, report the current understanding of causation, identify methods to assess this form of heart failure, and discuss current strategies for treatment.

DEFINITION AND TERMS

HFPEF has had other names over the years, including backward failure and diastolic heart failure. Although all three terms essentially describe the same group of patients, experts in the field of HF disagree as to the most correct term. Some experts have argued that diastolic HF is the more descriptive expression of the disease, reflecting more of the underlying pathophysiology, while others counter that such a term assumes too much given our still limited understanding. For now, HFPEF has become the more favored

J.D. Bisognano et al. (eds.), *Manual of Heart Failure Management*,
DOI: 10.1007/978-1-84882-185-9_5, © Springer-Verlag London Limited 2009

term because of the lack of consistent, widely-accepted diagnostic criteria, the difficulty in measuring diastolic function, and our imprecise knowledge of the mechanisms of this disorder.[5,6]

Regardless of the type, HF is a clinical syndrome. The modern definition was set forth by McKee et al.[7] in an observational study published in 1971, which codified a set of diagnostic criteria to evaluate and report on patients with HF from the Framingham Heart Study (Table 5.1). HF was defined as two major, or one major and two minor criteria.

As our understanding of HF improved and differences in prognosis and treatment became apparent, so did the importance of identifying those HF patients with and without preserved ejection fraction. In the late 1990s, the European Society of Cardiology defined HFPEF as signs or symptoms of HF in the presence of a normal or near normal left ventricular ejection fraction (LVEF > 45%) with diastolic dysfunction evidenced by abnormal left ventricular (LV) relaxation, filling, distensibility, or stiffness.[8,9] Because this definition required objective evidence of diastolic dysfunction, either by heart catheterization or echocardiography, its usefulness was limited by the availability of these modalities

TABLE 5.1. Diagnostic criteria of congestive heart failure

Major criteria

Orthopnea
Paroxysmal nocturnal dyspnea
Neck vein distention
Rales
Cardiomegaly
Pulmonary edema
S3 gallop
Increased venous pressure > 16 cm water
Circulation time > 25 sec
Hepatojugular reflux
Weight loss definitely in response to treatment

Minor criteria

Ankle edema
Nocturnal cough
Dyspnea on exertion
Hepatomegaly
Pleural effusion
Vital capacity decreased one-third from maximum
Tachycardia
Weight loss probably in response to treatment

and the accuracy and precision of measurement, which can be operator and reader dependent.

In 2000, Vasan and Levy[10] proposed a new classification system of diastolic HF, which did not absolutely require objective evidence of diastolic function, and instead, placed patients with the suspected diagnosis in one of three categories (definite, probable, and possible) based on the availability of objective LV and diastolic function assessment. However, this classification system was not widely adopted.

Presently, the term HFPEF describes a person who has signs and symptoms of HF and a preserved ejection fraction. Diastolic dysfunction is not required to make the diagnosis, even though it may be a common cause or contributing factor. HF with or without preserved ejection fraction is a clinical diagnosis; however, if an alternative explanation for the patient's symptoms can be made, such as a primary pulmonary pathology, this must be explored.[11-14]

Epidemiology

By the year 2040, it is estimated that the United States will have 77.2 million people 65 years of age or older, which will be 20.5% of the population.[15] Over 5 million people in the United States are currently diagnosed with HF, which is the most frequent cause of hospitalization in patients over the age of 65. Survival five years after the diagnosis of HF has improved from 43% in 1979–1984 to 52% in 1996–2000. However, the survival gains occurred more in men and younger people, less in women and the elderly.[1,16]

HF is the only major cardiovascular disorder on the rise in the United States.[17] The number of patients with HFPEF is increasing, and it is now reported to be as common as systolic HF (SHF).[18] In a study of all hospitalized patients with decompensated HF from 1987–2001 in Olmstead County, the prevalence of HFPEF increased from 38% to 54%. This increase was significant in both community-based and referral patients, and occurred without an increase in admissions of patients with SHF. Although the survival of patients with SHF increased over this 15-year period, the survival of those with HFPEF did not.[2]

The disease processes seem to affect slightly different populations. Elevated systolic blood pressure and atrial fibrillation tend to occur more commonly in patients with HFPEF, whereas atherosclerotic disease and myocardial infarction are more common in patients with SHF. HFPEF patients are also typically older, female and more often diagnosed in the out-patient setting. On an average, they have a lower New York Heart Association class (II vs. III) but interestingly have been found to have a significantly higher number of functional limitations at follow-up.[17–22]

More than 80% of HF admissions occur in patients > 65-years old.[17] Readmission rates are frequent and traditionally thought to occur more often in SHF. But, some studies now show no statistical difference in readmission rates between HFPEF and SHF, despite more digoxin use in HFPEF patients. A similar length of hospital stay has been found as well.[19,20]

Although there are conflicting data, mortality may be higher in patients with SHF. In a study at Washington University Medical Center, HF admissions in patients ≥70 years of age were examined. The mortality rate of SHF was found to be 23.2% at three months and 38.2% at one year compared with 13.5% at three months and 28.1% at one year in patients with HFPEF.[17] Similarly by six months, all-cause mortality was shown to be 13% for HFPEF and 21% for SHF in 413 patients studied prospectively at Yale-New Haven Hospital.[20] Mortality improves with increasing ejection fraction (EF) up to ~45%. For each 10% reduction in EF below 45%, the risk for all-cause mortality increases by up to 39%.[21] However, compared with matched controls, HFPEF patients still have up to a fourfold increased mortality risk.[18]

PATHOPHYSIOLOGY

Diastole is divided into four phases: isovolumic relaxation, early rapid diastolic filling, diastasis, and late diastolic filling secondary to atrial contraction. At the cellular level, repolarization causes the cardiomyocyte to relax by the reuptake of calcium back into the sarcoplasmic reticulum via an energy-dependent process. When repolarization begins, calcium dissociates from the troponin I/T/C complex, and a conformation change occurs. The troponin I/T/C complex and the abutting tropomyosin then block myosin heads from binding to the active site on actin, thus ending muscle contraction. The cardiomyocyte then returns to its resting shape given its viscoelastic properties. Diastole ends when the cardiomyocyte is again depolarized, calcium is extruded from the sarcoplasmic reticulum and binds with the troponin I/T/C complex, allowing the tropomyosin to move from the active actin-binding site and allowing the myosin heads to interact and move up the actin fibrils causing muscle contraction.[23]

The predominant abnormality of HFPEF is elevated end-diastolic filling pressure due to increased passive stiffness and impaired relaxation. At the macroscopic level, patients with HFPEF typically have concentric LV hypertrophy with increased wall thickness and mass, and an elevated mass to volume ratio.

This change in the LV geometry increases passive stiffness, leading to reduced compliance, elevating filling pressures, and ultimately abnormal filling of the left ventricle or "diastolic dysfunction."[14] In contrast to systolic failure in which LV end-diastolic volume is increased, LV volume is typically within the normal range or even reduced in patients with HFPEF. In addition, stroke volume and cardiac index have been found to be lower when compared with hypertensive controls, despite a normal EF.[24] Even in the setting of systolic blood pressure < 140, patients with LV hypertrophy will have reduced stroke volume index and cardiac index compared with those patients without LV hypertrophy.[25] This reduced stroke volume and cardiac index in HFPEF results in severe exercise intolerance with marked increase in pulmonary pressures at peak exercise, which can explain the dyspnea on exertion and perhaps the symptoms of chronic fatigue.[26]

At the microscopic level, abnormalities of calcium homeostasis, reduction of the ATP/ADP ratio, and changes in the cytoskeleton and extracellular matrix constitution and geometry also contribute to diastolic dysfunction.[27] The cardiomyocytes of HFPEF patients have been shown to have almost twice the resting tension of normal patients at the same sarcomere length. This finding is thought to be due to a reduction in sarcomere protein phosphoralation. In addition, a higher collagen volume fraction is found outside the myocytes, suggesting that there may be an imbalance of matrix metalloproteinases and their tissue inhibitors, resulting in decreased extracellular matrix degradation.[28–30] Compared with the myocardial structure in SHF, cardiomyocytes in HFPEF have increased diameter and passive force. Cardiomyocytes of SHF have equal collagen volume fraction and less myofibrillary density.[31] Reduction in the absolute ATP and ATP/ADP ratio, which also occurs in advanced HF, is thought to contribute to diastolic dysfunction as cardiomyocyte relaxation is an energy-dependent process requiring the use of ATP to reuptake calcium ions into the sarcoplasmic reticulum so that the myosin heads will detach from the actin filaments.[32]

Other postulated causes of HFPEF include increased systolic-vascular stiffening and cardiac volume overload. Although increases in resistive and pulsatile components of vascular load have been demonstrated in patients with HFPEF compared with normal patients, the findings are not significantly different from patients with hypertension.[24] Studies that have demonstrated the existence of patients with increased LV volume and end-diastolic pressure without impairments in diastolic filling are small, and have not been validated in larger series.[33] Worsening diastolic dysfunction seems to be the common pathway in the majority of HFPEF patients studied, but certainly may not be the only inciting cause.

ASSESSMENT

The signs and symptoms of HFPEF are similar to those in patients with SHF. Volume overload is a frequent problem and dyspnea, orthopnea, and rales occur with comparable frequency in both groups, although cardiomegaly and the frequency of the S3 occur less commonly in HFPEF. Also, HFPEF patients are more likely to have a lower New York Heart Association class.[19] Although there is often symptom overlap, the presentation of HFPEF tends to be different. Patients with SHF frequently present with signs of hypoperfusion, while patients with HFPEF typically do not. In fact, many patients with HFPEF present with uncontrolled hypertension or hypertensive urgency as the precipitant of their symptoms.

Pressure and volume measurements obtained from the gold-standard of cardiac catheterization are impractical in assessing HFPEF. Noninvasive methods can be utilized, such as echocardiography.[23] Echocardiography is very useful for the evaluation of LV systolic and diastolic function. Diastolic function is assessed using transmitral inflow velocity, isovolumic relaxation time, and deceleration time with pulse-wave Doppler. In addition, mitral annular velocity can be measured with tissue Doppler.[23,34]

During diastole, the majority of blood enters the left ventricle during the early rapid filling phase prior to atrial contraction. The ratio of the E (early filling) and A (atrial contraction) waves, measured on pulse-wave Doppler through the mitral valve, allows for a rudimentary assessment of diastolic function (Figure 5.1). A normal E/A ratio is 1–1.5. As diastolic dysfunction worsens, higher LV filling pressures make the heart more dependent on atrial contraction for diastolic filling since the passive gradient between the atrium and the ventricle is reduced, and early filling is less robust. This translates into a reversal in the normal E/A pattern and a reduction in the ratio to < 1. In addition, there is a deceleration of mitral inflow, and the mitral E wave deceleration time will initially prolong to > 230 ms. Isovolumic relaxation time, which is the time between aortic valve closure and mitral valve opening, is also prolonged to > 110 ms in the initial phase of abnormal relaxation. As diastolic dysfunction continues to worsen, atrial pressure rises in response to the elevated ventricular filling pressure. This change essentially restores the atrioventricular gradient and normalizes the E and the A filling pattern creating a "pseudonormal" E/A ratio, deceleration time, and isovolumic

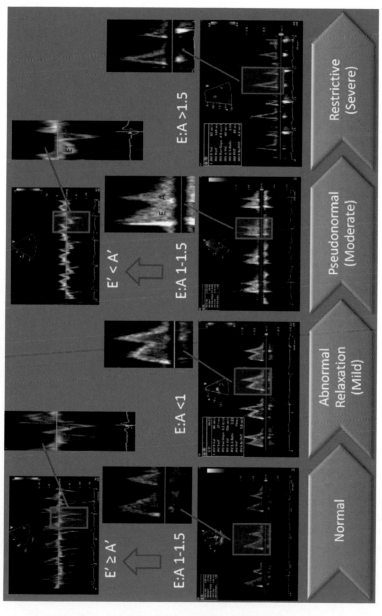

FIGURE 5.1.   Tissue doppler and mitral inflow doppler tracings from patients with varying degrees of diastolic dysfunction.

relaxation time. To recognize when the E/A ratio represents a normal filling pattern versus a "pseudonormal" filling pattern, tissue Doppler imaging can be utilized. Tissue Doppler imaging records the myocardial velocity during diastole. Similar to the transmitral flow velocities, the movement of the heart muscle can be recorded during early rapid filling and atrial contraction (E' and A'). The E'/A' ratio is usually > 1. When E/A ratio is normal and the E'/A' ratio is < 1, moderate to severe diastolic dysfunction is present.[34] Lastly, as diastolic dysfunction becomes severe, the E/A ratio will be > 1.5 with a deceleration time < 160 ms. The heart at this point takes on a more restrictive physiology.[3,9]

Other imaging modalities can assess for diastolic dysfunction but are not as routinely used. Nuclear scans (radionuclide angiograms) utilizing tagged red blood cells can measure indices of diastolic dysfunction, including the peak LV filling rate normalized to end-diastolic volume and the duration of isovolumic relaxation. Unfortunately, left atrial to left ventricular pressure gradients, as well as simultaneous pressure and volume changes of these chambers, are not able to be measured, which limits some of the utility of this method. Diastolic functional assessment by MRI and CT is being developed but remains experimental at this point.[23]

TREATMENT

Few well-designed (randomized, double-blind, placebo-controlled) studies exist examining targeted therapies for HFPEF. Studies are mostly small and some contradictory. Treatment at this point is based primarily on expert opinion and should be directed toward alleviating symptoms, treating known etiologies, and reversing the pathology caused by known etiologies (Figure 5.2).[13,27,35]

To improve symptoms, one of the key treatments is reducing pulmonary venous pressure. This can be achieved through a low salt diet and fluid restriction, and/or through diuretics and nitrates (which act to reduce central blood volume). ACE inhibitors, angiotensin receptor blockers (ARBs), or aldosterone antagonists also help prevent fluid from accumulating by blocking neurohumeral activation.[27] This benefit of ARBs impacts hospital admissions and exercise performance. In the CHARM-Preserved trial, candesartan was shown to significantly decrease the number of hospital admissions, although cardiovascular mortality was unchanged.[22] Blood pressure, when elevated, can also impair diastolic performance. Losartan has been shown to improve exercise performance of those HFPEF patients with a hypertensive response to exercise.[36] Tachycardia may exacerbate HFPEF symptoms, and, if present, needs to be treated. As the heart beats faster, there is less time

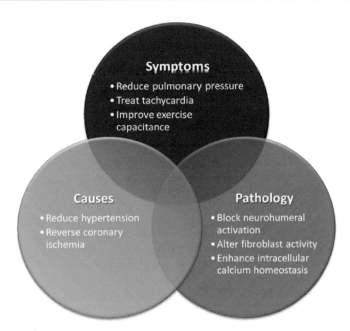

FIGURE 5.2. Treatment of HFPEF.

for the heart to relax, which results in higher filling pressures, and subsequently higher pulmonary pressures creating the signs and symptoms of HF. Tachycardia can also increase the myocardial oxygen demand further delaying relaxation, as relaxation is an energy-dependent process. Aerobic exercise in moderation may improve cardiovascular function and reduce the heart rate. Tachycardia can also be treated with beta blockers and nondihydropyridine calcium channel blockers.[27] Verapamil, in specific, has been shown in a small study to statistically improve peak filling rate as well as exercise capacity of HFPEF patients.[37] If tachycardia is present in the setting of atrial fibrillation or flutter, cardioversion to a sinus rhythm may improve symptoms by providing additional atrial preload.[13]

Common underlying etiologies of HFPEF include hypertension, coronary artery disease, and valvular heart disease. Less commonly, hypertrophic cardiomyopathy and infiltrative diseases such as cardiac amylodosis are involved. Evidence does exist that treating hypertension will reduce the incidence of developing HF.[38] In the setting of coronary artery disease, expert opinion considers coronary revascularization reasonable if demonstrable ischemia is thought to be contributing to cardiac dysfunction.[13]

In addition to alleviating symptoms and treating causes of HFPEF, finding pharmaceuticals that reverse pathology is a high priority. For instance, in addition to reducing fluid retention, blocking neurohumeral activation may reduce fibrosis by altering fibroblast activity or may improve calcium reuptake and ventricular relaxation through intracellular calcium modulation.[27] In HFPEF patients already receiving a stable dose of diuretics whose blood pressures were controlled to goal, the addition of enalapril showed statistical improvements in LV mass, diastolic filling parameters, and treadmill exercise time.[39] After a year of losartan therapy, hypertensive patients with biopsy-proven increased myocardial fibrosis had decreased chamber stiffness and collagen volume fraction.[30] Other classes of drugs that block neurohumeral activation have shown benefit as well. Propranolol can reduce total mortality up to 35% and total mortality plus nonfatal myocardial infarction up to 37% in HFPEF patients with a history of myocardial infarction who are already on diuretics and ACE inhibitors.[40] Because aldosterone antagonism has known benefits in SHF[41] and also blocks neurohumeral activation potentially reversing cardiac fibrosis, large ongoing studies are in progress examining the use of spironolactone in HFPEF, such as the Treatment of Reserved Cardiac Function Heart Failure with an Aldosterone Antagonist (TOPCAT) trial.[42]

SUMMARY

HFPEF is increasingly being identified as a cause of HF, and the prevalence is likely to increase as our population ages. The cause is multifactorial and poorly understood, and the lack of a consistent and widely accepted definition has hindered research. Echocardiography is particularly useful in helping to make the diagnosis. Treatment should focus on targeting symptoms, identifying and treating underlying etiologies, and attempting to reverse known pathologic processes.

References

1. Rosamond, W., et al., *Heart disease and stroke statistics–2007 update: a report from the American Heart Association Statistics Committee and Stroke Statistics Subcommittee*. Circulation, 2007. 115(5): pp. e69–e171.
2. Owan, T.E., et al., *Trends in prevalence and outcome of heart failure with preserved ejection fraction*. N Engl J Med, 2006. 355(3): pp. 251–9.
3. Haney, S., D. Sur, and Z. Xu, *Diastolic heart failure: a review and primary care perspective*. J Am Board Fam Pract, 2005. 18(3): pp. 189–98.
4. Banerjee, P., et al., *Diastolic heart failure: neglected or misdiagnosed?* J Am Coll Cardiol, 2002. 39(1): pp. 138–41.

5. Zile, M.R., *Heart failure with preserved ejection fraction: is this diastolic heart failure?* J Am Coll Cardiol, 2003. 41(9): pp. 1519–22.

6. Burkhoff, D., M.S. Maurer, and M. Packer, *Heart failure with a normal ejection fraction: is it really a disorder of diastolic function?* Circulation, 2003. 107(5): pp. 656–8.

7. McKee, P.A., et al., *The natural history of congestive heart failure: the Framingham study.* N Engl J Med, 1971. 285(26): pp. 1441–6.

8. *Guidelines for the diagnosis of heart failure. The Task Force on Heart Failure of the European Society of Cardiology.* Eur Heart J, 1995. 16(6): pp. 741–51.

9. *How to diagnose diastolic heart failure. European Study Group on Diastolic Heart Failure.* Eur Heart J, 1998. 19(7): pp. 990–1003.

10. Vasan, R.S. and D. Levy, *Defining diastolic heart failure: a call for standardized diagnostic criteria.* Circulation, 2000. 101(17): pp. 2118–21.

11. Zile, M.R., et al., *Heart failure with a normal ejection fraction: is measurement of diastolic function necessary to make the diagnosis of diastolic heart failure?* Circulation, 2001. 104(7): pp. 779–82.

12. Caruana, L., et al., *Do patients with suspected heart failure and preserved left ventricular systolic function suffer from "diastolic heart failure" or from misdiagnosis? A prospective descriptive study.* BMJ, 2000. 321(7255): pp. 215–8.

13. Hunt, S.A., *ACC/AHA 2005 guideline update for the diagnosis and management of chronic heart failure in the adult: a report of the American College of Cardiology/American Heart Association Task Force on Practice Guidelines (Writing Committee to Update the 2001 Guidelines for the Evaluation and Management of Heart Failure).* J Am Coll Cardiol, 2005. 46(6): pp. e1–e82.

14. Baicu, C.F., et al., *Left ventricular systolic performance, function, and contractility in patients with diastolic heart failure.* Circulation, 2005. 111(18): pp. 2306–12.

15. Redfield, M.M., *Heart failure-an epidemic of uncertain proportions.* N Engl J Med, 2002. 347(18): pp. 1442–4.

16. Roger, V.L., et al., *Trends in heart failure incidence and survival in a community-based population.* JAMA, 2004. 292(3): pp. 344–50.

17. Pernenkil, R., et al., *Course and prognosis in patients > or = 70 years of age with congestive heart failure and normal versus abnormal left ventricular ejection fraction.* Am J Cardiol, 1997. 79(2): pp. 216–9.

18. Vasan, R.S., et al., *Congestive heart failure in subjects with normal versus reduced left ventricular ejection fraction: prevalence and mortality in a population-based cohort.* J Am Coll Cardiol, 1999. 33(7): pp. 1948–55.

19. Hogg, K., K. Swedberg, and J. McMurray, *Heart failure with preserved left ventricular systolic function; epidemiology, clinical characteristics, and prognosis.* J Am Coll Cardiol, 2004. 43(3): pp. 317–27.

20. Smith, G.L., et al., *Outcomes in heart failure patients with preserved ejection fraction: mortality, readmission, and functional decline.* J Am Coll Cardiol, 2003. 41(9): pp. 1510–8.

21. Solomon, S.D., et al., *Influence of ejection fraction on cardiovascular outcomes in a broad spectrum of heart failure patients.* Circulation, 2005. 112(24): pp. 3738–44.

22. Yusuf, S., et al., *Effects of candesartan in patients with chronic heart failure and preserved left-ventricular ejection fraction: the CHARM-Preserved Trial.* Lancet, 2003. 362(9386): pp. 777–81.

23. Zipes, D.P. and E. Braunwald, *Braunwald's heart disease: a textbook of cardiovascular medicine.* 7th ed. 2005, Philadelphia, Pa.: Elsevier Saunders.

24. Lam, C.S., et al., *Cardiac structure and ventricular-vascular function in persons with heart failure and preserved ejection fraction from Olmsted County, Minnesota.* Circulation, 2007. 115(15): pp. 1982–90.

25. Aurigemma, G.P., et al., *Reduced left ventricular systolic pump performance and depressed myocardial contractile function in patients > 65 years of age with normal ejection fraction and a high relative wall thickness.* Am J Cardiol, 1995. 76(10): pp. 702–5.

26. Kitzman, D.W., et al., *Exercise intolerance in patients with heart failure and preserved left ventricular systolic function: failure of the Frank-Starling mechanism.* J Am Coll Cardiol, 1991. 17(5): pp. 1065–72.

27. Zile, M.R. and D.L. Brutsaert, *New concepts in diastolic dysfunction and diastolic heart failure: Part II: causal mechanisms and treatment.* Circulation, 2002. 105(12): pp. 1503–8.

28. Borbely, A., et al., *Cardiomyocyte stiffness in diastolic heart failure.* Circulation, 2005. 111(6): pp. 774–81.

29. Ahmed, S.H., et al., *Matrix metalloproteinases/tissue inhibitors of metalloproteinases: relationship between changes in proteolytic determinants of matrix composition and structural, functional, and clinical manifestations of hypertensive heart disease.* Circulation, 2006. 113(17): pp. 2089–96.

30. Diez, J., et al., *Losartan-dependent regression of myocardial fibrosis is associated with reduction of left ventricular chamber stiffness in hypertensive patients.* Circulation, 2002. 105(21): pp. 2512–7.

31. van Heerebeek, L., et al., *Myocardial structure and function differ in systolic and diastolic heart failure.* Circulation, 2006. 113(16): pp. 1966–73.

32. Neubauer, S., *The failing heart-an engine out of fuel.* N Engl J Med, 2007. 356(11): pp. 1140–51.

33. Maurer, M.S., et al., *Left heart failure with a normal ejection fraction: identification of different pathophysiologic mechanisms.* J Card Fail, 2005. 11(3): pp. 177–87.

34. Otto, C.M., *Textbook of clinical echocardiography.* 3rd ed. 2004, Philadelphia, Pa.: Elsevier Saunders. xiii, 541 p.

35. Aurigemma, G.P. and W.H. Gaasch, *Clinical practice. Diastolic heart failure.* N Engl J Med, 2004. 351(11): pp. 1097–105.

36. Warner, J.G., Jr., et al., *Losartan improves exercise tolerance in patients with diastolic dysfunction and a hypertensive response to exercise.* J Am Coll Cardiol, 1999. 33(6): pp. 1567–72.

37. Setaro, J.F., et al., *Usefulness of verapamil for congestive heart failure associated with abnormal left ventricular diastolic filling and normal left ventricular systolic performance.* Am J Cardiol, 1990. 66(12): pp. 981–6.

38. Kostis, J.B., et al., *Prevention of heart failure by antihypertensive drug treatment in older persons with isolated systolic hypertension. SHEP Cooperative Research Group*. JAMA, 1997. 278(3): pp. 212–6.

39. Aronow, W.S. and I. Kronzon, *Effect of enalapril on congestive heart failure treated with diuretics in elderly patients with prior myocardial infarction and normal left ventricular ejection fraction*. Am J Cardiol, 1993. 71(7): pp. 602–4.

40. Aronow, W.S., C. Ahn, and I. Kronzon, *Effect of propranolol versus no propranolol on total mortality plus nonfatal myocardial infarction in older patients with prior myocardial infarction, congestive heart failure, and left ventricular ejection fraction > or = 40% treated with diuretics plus angiotensin-converting enzyme inhibitors*. Am J Cardiol, 1997. 80(2): pp. 207–9.

41. Pitt, B., et al., *The effect of spironolactone on morbidity and mortality in patients with severe heart failure. Randomized Aldactone Evaluation Study Investigators*. N Engl J Med, 1999. 341(10): pp. 709–17.

42. Bernal, J., S.R. Pitta, and D. Thatai, *Role of the renin-angiotensin-aldosterone system in diastolic heart failure: potential for pharmacologic intervention*. Am J Cardiovasc Drugs, 2006. 6(6): pp. 373–81.

Chapter 6
Valvular Heart Failure

Ryan J. Hoefen and Eugene Storozynsky

When valvular dysfunction is the underlying cause of heart failure, its identification permits directed medical and/or surgical treatment that can change patient morbidity and mortality by improving patient symptoms and cardiac function. Thus, its prompt identification is important when evaluating a patient with new or worsening heart failure. The nature of the clinical presentation and cardiac dysfunction varies depending on the valve involved, its defect, and the precipitating cause. Here, we attempt to help readers understand the mechanism for heart failure that accompanies the various forms of valvular disease and its correlation with the clinical presentation. We will also outline the major underlying causes, physical exam findings, diagnostic testing, and treatment for each of the major forms of valvular dysfunction (summarized in table 6.1).

AORTIC STENOSIS

Aortic stenosis (AS) is generally the result of inflammation with progressive calcification and fibrosis of the aortic leaflets. The most common cause is *age-related degenerative calcific AS*, which is a slowly progressive process of stenosis thought to be mediated by chronic inflammation similar to that of atherosclerosis within vessel walls. However, AS may occur in younger patients if they are predisposed to inflammatory changes by congenital abnormality (most commonly bicuspid aortic valves) or rheumatic disease.

As aortic valve area decreases, there is increasing resistance to forward flow and a pressure gradient between the left ventricle and the aorta. In the early stages, left ventricular systolic pressures increase to maintain a normal stroke volume. Chronically, this

J.D. Bisognano et al. (eds.), *Manual of Heart Failure Management*,
DOI: 10.1007/978-1-84882-185-9_6, © Springer-Verlag London Limited 2009

TABLE 6.1. Summary of common etiologies, physical findings, and treatment for various types of valvular dysfunction

	Most common etiology(s)	Cardiac morphology	Significant exam findings	Accepted interventions
Aortic stenosis	Age-related calcific	LV concentric hypertrophy	Pulsus parvus et tardus; paradoxic splitting of S2; systolic crescendo/decrescendo murmur at base transmitted to carotids	Aortic valve replacement; balloon valvoplasty
Aortic regurgitation	Aortic root dilatation	LV dilatation	Head bobbing, "water hammer" pulse, "pistol-shot" femoral bruit, decrescendo diastolic murmur at left sternal border	Aortic valve replacement; digitalis, salt restriction, diuresis, vasodilators, ACE inhibitors, nifedipine
Mitral stenosis	Rheumatic fever	LA enlargement	apical diastolic thrill, mitral opening snap during expiration, and rumbling diatolic murmur with patient in left lateral decub position	Balloon valvoplasty preferred over surgical valve repair or replacement
Mitral regurgitation	MV prolapse, ischemia, or any cause of LV dilatation	Massive LV enlargement and hypertrophy; LA enlargement	Loud apical holosystolic or decrescendo murmur radiating to axilla exacerbated by Valsalva or isometric exercise	Mitral valve replacement; vasodilators, sodium restriction, diuretics

Tricuspid Stenosis	Rheumatic disease	RA enlargement	Diastolic murmur at left sternal border accentuated by inspiration, decreased by expiration or Valsalva; ascites, peripheral edema	Intensive salt restriction and diuresis; valve may be replaced at the time of mitral valve surgery if there is concurrent mitral dysfunction
Tricuspid regurgitation	RV dilatation	RA and RV enlargement	Holosystolic murmur at left sternal border accentuated by inspiration and decreased by expiration or Valsalva	Treatment of underlying cause for RV dilatation
Pulmonic stenosis	Congenital defect	RV hypertrophy	Harsh crescendo/decrescendo systolic murmur at the upper left sternal border	Balloon valvoplasty preferred over surgical repair
Pulmonic regurgitation	Pulmonary hypertension, infective endocarditis	RV hypertrophy	Wide split S2, diastolic crescendo/decrescendo murmur at 3rd–4th intercostal space	Rarely required

results in concentric hypertrophy and, to a lesser extent, dilatation of the left ventricle. Patients are rarely symptomatic in the early stages.[10]

As aortic valve area decreases, there will eventually be physiologic decompensation that is accompanied by development of exertional dyspnea, angina pectoris, and syncope. A valve area less than 1 cm2 is generally considered to be "severe" stenosis, but the onset of symptoms is poorly predicted by valve area and can occur before or after this threshold is reached.[1] The thickening ventricle requires increased diastolic filling pressures, which are transmitted to the left atrium and pulmonary vasculature. This is exacerbated by tachycardia since decreased diastolic filling time requires even higher filling pressures, thus producing high pulmonary pressures and consequent dyspnea with exertion. Angina is the result of an inability to meet the increased oxygen demand required by the thick ventricle through vessels narrowed by the high transmural pressures and, often, concomitant atherosclerotic vessel disease. If cardiac contractility decreases or LV hypertrophy is insufficient to compensate for increasing afterload, cardiac output begins to decline. In this case, syncope may occur during exertion if the heart cannot generate the increased cardiac output required for sufficient cerebral perfusion in the setting of dilated vessels within exercising muscles. Prior to the wide availability of surgical valve repair or replacement, the mean amount of time between the first symptoms of AS and death was about three years, often occurring as a result of sudden cardiac death.[12]

Characteristic physical exam findings of AS include *pulsus parvus et tardus* (slowly rising pulse with a sustained peak), delayed aortic closure (aortic closure may occur simultaneous with or even after pulmonic closure, the latter of which is termed paradoxic splitting of the S2), and a low-pitched, rasping crescendo/decrescendo systolic murmur heard best at the heart base with transmission to the carotid arteries. As the valve area narrows, the murmur peaks later in systole. The murmur also may become softer as the valve area decreases. Other findings of AS are those typical of LV hypertrophy, including lateral displacement of the apical impulse, S4 heart sound, and accentuation of the venous *a* wave on inspection of the jugular veins.

Electrocardiography and chest radiography usually demonstrate only nonspecific findings of LV hypertrophy. However, as with other valve lesions, echocardiography is a very sensitive and specific method for detecting AS. With the use of Doppler imaging, the trans-valvular gradient and valve area can be estimated with good accuracy.

No medical treatment has been shown to be of benefit in the treatment of asymptomatic AS. Statins have been hypothesized to slow the progression of AS by decreasing inflammation within the valve, although clinical trials have failed to demonstrate any benefit thus far.[3]

The primary treatment for symptomatic AS is aortic valve replacement (AVR). Severe AS with symptoms and/or LV systolic dysfunction (ejection fraction less than 50%) is a Class I indications to perform AVR, as is the presence of severe AS in a patient who is undergoing CABG or surgery of the aorta or other heart valves according to an ACC/AHA panel of experts.[1] Patients who have critical AS without symptoms should be monitored with annual echocardiograms, and they undergo surgery if LV systolic dysfunction develops. Balloon valuloplasty is an alternative that is primarily used in children with congenital, non-calcific AS. In adults, there is a high rate of restenosis, so it is usually reserved for palliation or as a "bridge" to surgery in patients who are too ill to undergo surgery (ACC/AHA Class IIb indication[1]).

AORTIC REGURGITATION

Aortic regurgitation (AR) is due to a primary disorder of the aortic valve or the aortic root. Aortic root disease, which has become more common than primary valvular etiologies,[4] may be due to connective tissue disorders (Marfans or Ehlers-Danlos), severe hypertension, or retrograde aortic dissection. Primary valvular causes include rheumatic disease, rheumatoid spondylitis, and congenital abnormalities. Acute AR may occur as a result of infective endocarditis or trauma. AR can also occur with mixed AS, which is almost always due to rheumatic or congenital disease.

In AR, regurgitation of a portion of the total stroke volume with each heartbeat compromises the effective forward stroke volume. In chronic AR, the effective forward stroke volume is maintained by increasing the total stroke volume. This is primarily achieved by LV dilatation and eccentric hypertrophy.[7] In the early stage, these patients may experience palpitations in the chest or head, particularly with exertion, which may be quite uncomfortable for some. As LV dilatation progresses, the myocardium must generate increasing wall tension to maintain sufficient cardiac output. Eventually, the LV cannot maintain a sufficient effective forward stroke volume, particularly during exertion. As this occurs, cardiac output may be normal at rest, but fails to rise normally with exertion, producing exertional dyspnea. Late in the disease, elevation in diastolic LV pressure caused by regurgitant flow causes secondary elevation in LA, PA wedge, PA, and RV pressures. Patients may then complain of orthopnea, paroxysmal nocturnal dyspnea, and excessive diaphoresis. Finally, there may be insufficient resting cardiac output. In acute AR, the lack of compensatory LV dilatation results in quickly increased LV diastolic pressure resulting in elevated LA and PA pressures. Pulmonary edema and cardiogenic shock may occur quickly.

Ischemia may occur in these patients with longstanding AI even in the absence of coronary artery disease because oxygen demand is increased by LV dilatation and increased wall tension while coronary blood flow is reduced by suboptimal diastolic pressure. Thus, patients may have angina with exertion or at rest. In many cases, the angina does not respond to sublingual nitroglycerin.

Physical examination of patients with chronic, compensated AR may identify a widened pulse pressure. However, this may not be present in advanced or acute AI where there is elevated LV diastolic pressure and poor LV systolic function. Physical examination may also reveal bobbing of the head with systole or even jarring of the entire body. There is a heaving LV impulse that is displaced laterally and inferiorly. There may be a diastolic thrill at the left sternal border as well as a systolic thrill transmitted along the carotid arteries. A "water-hammer" (Corrigan's) pulse, abrupt distention and collaspse of the large arteries, is one of the most characteristic findings of AR. There may also be a loud "pistol-shot" sound over the femoral arteries (Traube's sign) as well as a "to-and-fro" murmur when slight compression is applied to the femoral artery with a stethocope (Duroziez's sign). Even capillary pulsation may be evident as alternate flushing and blanching at the root of the nail when pressure is applied at the tip (Quincke's pulse). Cardiac auscultation may reveal an absence of aortic closure, S3 and S4 sounds, and a high-pitched, blowing, decrescendo diastolic murmur along the left sternal border that becomes louder and longer as the disease progresses. The murmur is accentuated by sitting, leaning forward, with breath held in forced expiration. There may also be a loud systolic ejection murmur at the base of the heart transmitted to the carotids that is higher pitched and shorter than the murmur of AS. There may also be a soft, low-pitched, rumbling middiastolic bruit thought to be due to displacement of the anterior mitral valve leaflet by the AR jet (Austin Flint murmur). The features of AR are accentuated by hand grip due to increased systemic vascular resistance.

ECG usually shows LV hypertrophy and ST segment depression and T wave inversion (strain pattern). Severe disease may also lead to left axis deviation, as well as QRS prolongation due to extensive myocardial fibrosis. Echo is very sensitive for detecting AR and helpful in determining severity as well as helping to identify the cause or at least in differentiating primary valve vs. aortic root disorders.[1] Chest X-ray may show massive cardiomegaly. Catheterization should be done preoperatively to identify coexistant coronary disease.

Although surgery is the only definitive treatment, symptoms of heart failure can be improved with digitalis, salt restriction, diuretics, vasodilators, and ACE inhibitors. Long acting nifedipine has been shown to delay the need for surgery. Nitrates are typically not as helpful for angina as they are in ischemic cardiomyopathy, but may still provide some relief.

The key issue regarding surgery is that of timing. Since chronic AI progresses slowly, not all patients will require surgery. Rather, they should be monitored closely and generally followed by echocardiogram every six months. Surgery is generally indicated when there are either severe symptoms or LV dysfunction (EF < 55% or LV end-systolic volume > 55 ml/m^2). If surgery is delayed for too long, LV function may not recover significantly.

MITRAL STENOSIS

Mitral stenosis (MS) is the result of valve leaflets being thickened by fibrous tissue and/or calcium deposits. The disease progresses over time as the thickened leaflets become further calcified due to immobilization. This is nearly always caused by rheumatic fever, thus its incidence appears to be decreasing in developed countries.[2] It often coexists with mitral regurgitation, which is discussed below. Less common causes of MS include congenital defects, malignant carcinoid, systemic lupus erythematosus, and rheumatoid arthritis.

A normal mitral valve has an area of approximately 6 cm^2 and allows unimpeded flow from the left atrium to the left ventricle with essentially no pressure gradient between the two chambers. As the valve narrows to less than 2 cm^2, left atrial pressure increases as resistance to flow across the valve increases. The increased pressure gradient is exacerbated when heart rate increases since shortened diastole requires higher flow rates across the valve to achieve appropriate LV filling. As a result, patients may experience shortness of breath with exertion at this stage. Cardiac output may also fail to rise normally with exertion. Other causes of increased heart rate including emotional stress, thyrotoxicosis, and pregnancy can also produce symptoms. Similarly, as LA pressure produces progressive LA enlargement, there is a propensity to develop atrial fibrillation, which may hasten symptoms.

Critical stenosis of the mitral valve (<1 cm^2) requires approximately a 20 mmHg pressure gradient across the valve, resulting in significant pulmonary hypertension, right ventricular failure, and finally systemic venous congestion. This is accompanied by orthopnea, paroxysmal nocturnal dyspnea, and hemoptysis.[9] Cardiac output may become suboptimal at rest and may not rise (in fact, it may even worsen) with activity. Systemic emboli may complicate the late stage as atrial arrhythmias and increasing LA enlargement increase the risk of developing atrial thrombi.

Physical exam may reveal an apical diastolic thrill with the patient in left lateral decubitus position. Characteristic auscultatory findings include a mitral opening snap most audible during expiration medial to the cardiac apex followed by a low rumbling murmur at the apex with the patient in the left lateral decubitus position, then an accentuated, snapping, and slightly delayed S1 sound. Pulmonary hypertension may be apparent as a closely split or fixed S2 with an accentuated P2, and pulmonary systolic ejection click.

An EKG may only be remarkable for LA enlargement. If severe pulmonary hypertension is present, there may also be RA enlargement, right axis deviation, and RV hypertrophy. As with other forms of valvular dysfunction, echocardiogram is quite sensitive and specific for detecting MS.[2]

Medical treatment of MS is quite limited and is primarily aimed at treating complications of the disease. Sodium restriction and diuresis may improve symptoms of pulmonary congestion. Since atrial fibrillation exacerbates symptoms, cardioversion or rate control may provide some relief. Finally, long-term anticoagulation may be required in the event of thromboembolic complications.

Balloon valvotomy, the inflation of a balloon placed across the mitral valve, is the preferred method of valve repair because of lower morbidity and mortality. The balloon is placed at the valve by percutaneous right heart catheterization with septal puncture. This procedure is most successful if leaflets are thin and not calcified. It is contraindicated if there is moderate to severe mitral regurgitation or left atrial thrombus. It is primarily indicated in patients who are symptomatic or have moderate or severe valve stenosis with pulmonary hypertension (PA systolic pressure $>$ 50 mmHg or $>$ 60 mmHg during exercise).[11] Surgical valve repair may be required if balloon valvotomy is not possible, unsuccessful, or results in restenosis. Mitral valve replacement is also necessary if there is coexistent mitral regurg, the valve is damaged from a previous repair, or if the valve cannot be sufficiently repaired.

MITRAL REGURGITATION

The initial cause of mitral regurgitation (MR) may be mitral valve prolapse, rheumatic heart disease, congenital defects of the endocardial cushion, ischemia (either ischemic cardiomyopathy resulting in chronic MR or ischemia at the base of the papillary muscle causing acute or even intermittent MR), or LV dilatation of any cause resulting in enlargement of the mitral annulus. Acute causes of MR include ischemia, infectious endocarditis, and trauma. MR may complicate a myocardial infarction and should be suspected in patients recovering from MI who are found to have a new systolic murmur. Regardless of the initial cause, the disease is almost always progressive since MR results in LV and LA enlargement, which further prevent valve closure if there is accompanying dilatation of the mitral annulus.[5]

There are two primary mechanisms of physiologic decompensation in patients with MR. First, the regurgitant flow causes elevated LA pressure, which is transmitted to the pulmonary circulation, causing pulmonary congestion, edema, and, ultimately, right heart failure and systemic venous congestion. This process can occur rapidly in cases of acute MR. However, in chronic MR, LA compliance will often increase, preventing severe elevations in pulmonary pressures. Therefore, patients with longstanding MR are more prone to developing symptoms reflective of the second mechanism, which is reduction in effective cardiac output as a result of progressive LV dilatation and decreasing contractility. Since patients tend to have hyperdynamic LV function in the early stage of the disease to compensate for the regurgitation, even a mildly reduced EF can signify significant decompensation. These patients tend to present with fatigue due to poor cardiac output. LA enlargement in these patients nearly always results in atrial fibrillation.

On examination, S1 is usually absent, soft, or buried in the murmur. The murmur is typically a loud holosystolic or decrescendo apical murmur radiating to the axilla. The location of the murmur may vary depending on the direction of the regurgitant jet. It has been said to have a "cooing" quality if there is a flail leaflet. The murmur is exacerbated by isometric strain, such as Valsalva. The aortic valve may close prematurely, causing wide splitting of S2. There may also be an audible S3 and/or S4. Associated findings may include a palpable systolic thrill at the cardiac apex, which is often laterally displaced.

As with other types of valve dysfunction, electrocardiography may show only nonspecific findings, while echocardiography is very sensitive and specific for identifying MR. ECG may show LA or bi-atrial enlargement if there is sinus rhythm, although MR is often associated with atrial fibrillation. There are also likely to be high voltages consistent with LV enlargement. MR will be readily visualized on echocardiogram. 2D imaging can estimate LV function, and Doppler imaging can estimate the severity of regurgitation. Left heart catheterization can show regurgitation by the prompt appearance of contrast in the LA after injection into the LV. Catheterization should be performed in patients with planned surgical treatment to determine whether coronary bypass should be done at the same time.

Conservative treatment includes restricting physical activities that produce dyspnea/fatigue, reducing sodium intake, and enhancing sodium excretion with diuretics. Vasodilators may help increase forward cardiac output. ACE inhibitors are an excellent choice for chronic MR. Intravenous nitroprusside or nitroglycerin may be helpful in acute or severe MR. Anticoagulation and/or leg binders may help to prevent thromboembolic disease in late stages. Antibiotics may also be considered for endocarditis prophylaxis prior to high risk procedures in patients with MR, although the most recent AHA/ACC guidelines no longer consider this an absolute indication.

The only definitive treatment for mitral regurgitation is surgery. Asymptomatic or minimally symptomatic patients with normal LV function (EF > 60%) may remain stable for years and should not undergo surgery. However, if symptoms have a significant impact on the patient's lifestyle or there is LV dysfunction, surgical treatment should be offered, which may yield significant LV functional improvement.[6] In many cases, the mitral valve can be reconstructed or an annuloplasty ring may be placed, but valve replacement is often necessary. The valve may be replaced with a bioprosthetic or a mechanical bileaflet valve. Bioprosthetic valves are prone to late mechanical dysfunction while mechanical valves require lifelong anticoagulation therapy and thus are associated with risks of bleeding or thromboembolism. Therefore, careful consideration must be made in deciding which type of valve is most appropriate at the time of surgery.

TRICUSPID STENOSIS

Tricuspid stenosis (TS) is generally caused by rheumatic fever and only occurs in association with other valve lesions (generally MS). As the pressure gradient across the valve increases, so does the RA pressure, resulting in RA enlargement and systemic venous congestion. The decreased right heart output may decrease pulmonary pressures despite the presence of MS, thus improving symptoms of (or even masking) MS. Patients will typically complain of discomfort due to ascites and edema, as well as fatigue secondary to low CO. The diastolic murmur of TS is best heard along the left sternal border and is accentuated during inspiration due to increased flow across the valve and decreased during expiration and Valsalva maneuver. Intensive salt restriction and diuresis may improve symptoms of systemic venous congestion and improve surgical risk. Valve repair or replacement is typically carried out at the time of mitral valve surgery.[8]

TRICUSPID REGURGITATION

Tricuspid regurgitation (TR) is generally secondary to RV dilatation of any other cause, but can also be due to rheumatic fever, infarction of RV papillary muscles, tricuspid prolapse, infective endocarditis, trauma, or congenital defects. Its primary effects are systemic venous congestion and reduced cardiac output. Like TS, it can reduce the signs and symptoms of pulmonary hypertension. It produces a holosystolic murmur along the lower left sternal border that intensifies during inspiration and diminishes during expiration or Valsalva maneuver. Atrial fibrillation is usually present due to atrial enlargement. ECG usually shows RA and RV enlargement. Isolated TR in the absence of pulmonary hypertension (such as in infectious endocarditis or trauma) may be well-tolerated and not require further treatment. In many cases, TR may resolve if the underlying cause of RV enlargement is treated, such as surgical repair of a mitral valve when pulmonary hypertension causes RV enlargement. However, recovery may be speeded with tricuspid valvuloplasty. In cases of TR with severe valve deformity due to rheumatic disease, surgical valve repair or replacement should be carried out, particularly if there is no pulmonary hypertension (and hence little chance of improvement with correction of the underlying cause for pulmonary hypertension).[8]

PULMONIC VALVE DYSFUNCTION

Pulmonic valve dysfunction is far less common than the other forms of valvular disease described earlier. Regurgitation may result from infective endocarditis or dilatation of the pulmonic valve ring by severe pulmonary hypertension, but these are unlikely to be of hemodynamic consequence. Pulmonic stenosis is an uncommon congenital defect and may be progressive if the obstruction is moderate or severe leading to presentation in adulthood. The obstruction may limit flow sufficiently to prevent cardiac output from meeting metabolic demand during exertion, producing exertional dyspnea, fatigue, and syncope. The RV undergoes hypertrophy and a forceful atrial contraction is required for RV filling. If RV systolic pressures exceed that of the LV, right-to-left shunt may occur through a patent foramen ovale or atrial septal defect, resulting in cyanosis. On physical exam, the murmur of pulmonic stenosis is a harsh systolic crescendo-decrescendo sound at the upper left sternal border. The strong atrial contraction may be manifested by prominent *a* waves in the jugular venous pulse or even presystolic pulsation of the liver. The ECG may show right axis deviation, RV hypertrophy, and RA enlargement. Treatment is usually performed by balloon valvuloplasty, but may sometimes require surgical valve repair.

References

1. Bonow, R.O., B.A. Carabello, K. Chatterjee, A.C. de Leon, Jr, D.P. Faxon, M.D. Freed, W.H. Gaasch, B.W. Lytle, R.A. Nishimura, P.T. O'Gara, R.A. O'Rourke, C.M. Otto, P.M. Shah, and J.S. Shanewise. "ACC/AHA 2006 Guidelines for the Management of Patients with Valvular Heart Disease." Circulation. 2006; 114:e84-e231.
2. Carabello, B.A. "Modern management of mitral stenosis." Circulation. 2005; 112:432-437.
3. Cowell, S.J., D.E. Newby, R.J. Prescott, et al., "A randomized trial of intensive lipid-lowering therapy in calcific aortic stenosis." N Engl J Med 2005; 352:2389-2397.
4. Dare, A.J., J.P. Veinot, W.D. Edwards, H.D. Tazelaar, H.V. Schaff. "New observations on the etiology of aortic valve disease: a surgical pathologic study of 236 cases from 1990." Hum Pathol. 1993; 24:1330-1338.
5. Enriquez-Sarano, M., A.J. Basmadjian, A. Rossi, K.R. Bailey, J.B. Seward, and A.J. Tajik. "Progression of mitral regurgitation: a prospective Doppler echocardiographic study". J Am Coll Cardiol 1999; 34:1137-1144.
6. Enriquez-Sarano, M. "Timing of mitral valve surgery." Heart 2002; 87:79.
7. Grossman, W., D. Jones, and L.P. McLaurin. "Wall stress and patterns of hypertrophy in the human left ventricle". J Clin Invest 1975; 56:56-64.
8. Ha, J.W., N. Chung, Y. Jang, S.J. Rim. "Tricuspid stenosis and regurgitation: Doppler and color flow echocardiography and cardiac catheterization findings." Clin Cardio 2000; 23:51.
9. Hugenholtz, P.G., T.J. Ryan, S.W. Stein, and W.H. Belmann. "The spectrum of pure mitral stenosis. hemodynamicstudies in relation to clinical disability." Am J Cardiol. 1962; 10:773-784.
10. Krayenbuehl, H.P., O.M. Hess, M. Ritter, E.S. Monrad, and H. Hoppeler. "Left ventricular systolic function in aortic stenosis. Eur Heart J. 1988; 9 Suppl E:19-23.
11. Palacios, I.F., P.L. Sanchez, L.C. Harrell, A.E. Weyman, and P.C. Block. "Which patients benefit from percutaneous mitral balloon valvuloplasty? Prevalvuloplasty and postvalvuloplasty variables that predict long-term outcome." Circulation 2002; 105:1465-1471.
12. Ross, J. Jr. and E. Braunwald. "Aortic stenosis." Circulation. 1968; 38:61-67.

Chapter 7
Pharmacologic Therapy

Jennifer Falvey and Burns C. Blaxall

INTRODUCTION

The goals for therapy of symptomatic heart failure (HF) are ultimately to minimize risk factors, reduce symptoms, slow progression of the disease, and improve survival. Multiple interventions are available to the clinician, ranging from lifestyle modifications to surgical and device interventions. A host of clinical trials have demonstrated that careful pharmacologic management can achieve these goals in a majority of patients. The focus of this chapter will be to highlight such agents and provide recommendations for their use concordant with current recommendations from the American Heart Association and the American College of Cardiology (see Figure 7.1).

BETA BLOCKERS (β-ADRENERGIC RECEPTOR ANTAGONISTS)

Beta blockers have long been utilized to treat hypertension, angina, arrhythmias, coronary artery disease, and ischemia. More recently, beta blockers have produced uniformly beneficial effects in patients with HF from various causes and in all stages. This is due in large part to their inhibition of the harmful effects of chronic activation of the sympathetic nervous system, which is a hallmark of HF. Significant effects have included improvement in survival, morbidity, ejection fraction, quality of life, remodeling, hospitalization, and incidence of sudden death.

Beta blockers are indicated in all stable HF patients with left ventricular dysfunction unless contraindicated (see Figure 7.1).[1]

J.D. Bisognano et al. (eds.), *Manual of Heart Failure Management*,
DOI: 10.1007/978-1-84882-185-9_7, © Springer-Verlag London Limited 2009

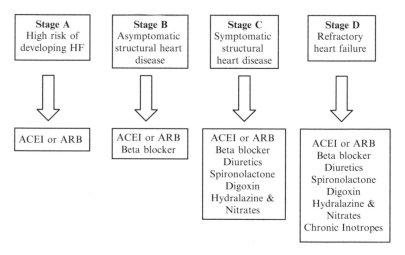

FIGURE 7.1. ACC/AHA heart failure stages and recommended therapies.

These agents should be initiated at a low dose and titrated slowly to doses proven to reduce mortality (see Table 7.1), to improve tolerability, and to limit adverse effects. Edema and fluid retention can be managed with the addition of a diuretic or by adjusting current diuretic therapy. Concurrent antihypertensive medications may need to be adjusted if hypotension occurs. Dosage may require reduction in patients who exhibit symptomatic bradycardia or fatigue. Withdrawal of therapy is not necessary in most cases. Abrupt withdrawal of therapy should be avoided to prevent acute worsening of symptoms.

Three agents in particular have demonstrated significant improvements over standard therapy in clinical trials involving patients with HF (bisoprolol, carvedilol, and metoprolol succinate XL). The CIBIS II trial enrolled stable patients with NYHA class III–IV symptoms (EF < 35%), who were already receiving an ACEI, to determine the effect of bisoprolol on mortality.[2] All-cause mortality was significantly reduced in the bisoprolol group compared to placebo, as were hospital readmissions and sudden death.

Carvedilol has been studied in thousands of HF patients, including one trial which showed a modest reduction in mortality compared to placebo.[3] There was also a significant reduction in the combined endpoint of death or time to first hospitalization. Unlike the other agents, which are beta-1 adrenergic receptor selective antagonists, carvedilol also possesses alpha-adrenergic

TABLE 7.1. Medications used in the treatment of heart failure

-	Initial daily dose	Maximum daily dose
Angiotensin converting enzyme inhibitors		
Captopril	6.25 mg three times daily	50 mg three times daily
Enalapril	2.5 mg twice daily	10–20 mg twice daily
Fosinopril	5–10 mg daily	40 mg daily
Lisinopril	2.5–5 mg daily	40 mg daily
Quinapril	5 mg twice daily	20 mg twice daily
Ramipril	1.25–2.5 mg daily	10 mg daily
Trandolapril	1 mg daily	4 mg daily
Angiotensin II receptor blockers		
Candesartan	4–8 mg daily	32 mg daily
Valsartan	20–40 mg twice daily	160 mg twice daily
Aldosterone receptor blockers		
Eplerenone	25 mg daily	50 mg daily
Spironolactone	12.5–25 mg daily	25 mg daily
Beta blockers		
Bisoprolol	1.25 mg daily	10 mg daily
Carvedilol	3.125 mg twice daily	25–50 mg twice daily
Metoprolol succinate	12.5–25 mg daily	200 mg daily
Vasodilators		
Hydralazine	25–37.5 mg three times daily	75–100 mg three times daily
Isosorbide dinitrate	10–20 mg three times daily	40 mg three times daily
Isosorbide mononitrate	30 mg daily	120 mg daily
Cardiac glycosides		
Digoxin	0.125–0.25 mg daily	N/A

*Carvedilol 50 mg twice daily indicated in patients >85 kg.
**Target serum digoxin concentrations: 0.5–1 ng/L.

receptor blocking effects. Metoprolol succinate XL has also been shown to reduce all-cause mortality compared to placebo in patients with NYHA class II–IV (EF < 40%) who were already receiving standard therapy.[4]

Although it is unclear which beta blocker is superior both in general and in particular etiologies, beta-blocker therapy is clearly a therapeutically valuable tool in the HF armamentarium.

THE RENIN–ANGIOTENSIN–ALDOSTERONE SYSTEM

Inhibiting the deleterious effects of the Renin–Angiotensin-Aldosterone System (RAAS) is a primary area of focus in the prevention and the treatment of HF. Vasoconstriction, sodium and water retention, aldosterone release, ventricular remodeling, and myocardial hypertrophy are well-known detrimental consequences of excessive circulating angiotensin II. A number of current medications target different points of the RAAS to attenuate these effects, including angiotensin converting enzyme inhibitors (ACEI), angiotensin II receptor antagonists (ARBs), and aldosterone receptor antagonists.

ANGIOTENSIN CONVERTING ENZYME INHIBITORS

These agents inhibit angiotensin II generation by blocking the enzyme responsible for conversion of angiotensin I to angiotensin II. Kininase is also inhibited by ACEI producing elevations in the vasodilator bradykinin, as well as other vasodilating prostaglandins. Long-term ACEI therapy improves cardiac index (CI), stroke volume (SV), systemic vascular resistance (SVR), and mean arterial pressure (MAP).

The beneficial effects of ACEI have been studied in thousands of patients with varying etiologies and stages of HF. ACEI have proven to reduce mortality and hospitalizations and improve clinical status in numerous placebo-controlled trials. The SOLVD trial evaluated enalapril in patients receiving conventional HF therapy (diuretics and digoxin), and demonstrated a 16% relative risk reduction in mortality.[5] Enalapril was also studied against an active comparator group of hydralazine and isosorbide dinitrate (ISDN), where it significantly reduced mortality.[1]

ACEI should be prescribed to all patients with left ventricular dysfunction regardless of symptoms unless contraindicated (see Figure 7.1).[1] Patients at high risk of developing HF should also be considered candidates. High risk patients include those with hypertension, diabetes, atherosclerosis, obesity, or metabolic syndrome. Typically, ACEI are used in combination with beta blockers and potentially with diuretics if volume overload is exhibited.

Therapy should be initiated at low doses and titrated gradually to doses proven to reduce mortality (see Table 7.1). Caution should be exercised in patients with hypotension, hyperkalemia, bilateral renal artery stenosis, or renal insufficiency at baseline. Renal function and serum potassium must be monitored closely after initiation and routinely during therapy. Hyperkalemia associated with ACEI therapy may be managed by adjusting the dosage of or discontinuing potassium-sparing diuretics and/or potassium supplements. Maintaining appropriate fluid status, usually with diuretic therapy, is essential to reduce azotemia and obtain maximal therapeutic benefit.

A dry, nonproductive cough is frequently associated with ACEI therapy and can be attributed to kinin accumulation. Patients should be urged to continue therapy, if tolerable. An alternative ACEI should be attempted prior to substitution with an ARB. A rare, but well-known, risk associated with ACEI therapy is angioedema. This life-threatening adverse reaction is most commonly acute in onset but may occur late in therapy. Re-exposure to ACEI is not recommended, therefore alternative therapies such as hydralazine and ISDN should be considered. Angioedema has also been associated with ARBs, thus switching from an ACEI should be done with extreme caution.[6]

Nonsteroidal anti-inflammatory drugs (NSAIDs) cause vasoconstriction of the afferent arterioles resulting in a decrease in intraglomerular pressure and glomerular filtration rate. Hence, NSAIDs should be avoided in patients with HF, particularly those taking ACEI.

ANGIOTENSIN RECEPTOR BLOCKERS

Angiotensin receptor blockers (ARBs) are an appealing option in patients who are intolerant to the cough associated with ACEIs. Cough is less prevalent with ARB therapy as kinin production is unaffected by angiotensin II receptor antagonism. Blocking the RAAS at the receptor level will antagonize angiotensin II activity regardless of the production pathway.

ARB therapy is considered an alternative to first line ACEI therapy due to fewer randomized, controlled trials in patients with HF. Several clinical trials have illustrated a reduction in morbidity and mortality in patients with left ventricular dysfunction.

The ELITE II trial demonstrated that the ARB losartan is not superior to the ACEI captopril in reducing all-cause mortality in patients with symptomatic HF (EF < 40%), and produced less adverse reactions, such as cough.[7] The Val-HeFT trial studied patients with NYHA class II–IV already receiving an ACEI and/or beta blocker and found there was no significant reduction in all-cause mortality between the two groups.[8]

The CHARM trials evaluated the ARB candesartan in patients with NYHA class II–IV, EF < 40%, with or without concurrent ACEI therapy, and found a reduction in cardiovascular death or hospital admissions due to HF in the candesartan group.[9] Valsartan was studied in post-myocardial infarction patients with left ventricular dysfunction with or without symptomatic HF and was considered noninferior to captopril in reducing mortality in this population.[10] The combination group of valsartan and captopril exhibited a higher rate of hypotension and renal dysfunction compared to the captopril group.

ARBs should be considered in all patients with left ventricular dysfunction or at high risk for developing HF, if intolerant to ACEI (see Figure 7.1).[1] Patients who have not previously shown intolerance to ACEI should not be initiated on ARBs until proven intolerant. These agents should not be considered alternatives to ACEI in patients who have developed hypotension, angioedema, renal dysfunction, or hyperkalemia as these effects can still occur with ARB therapy.

Similar to ACEI therapy, ARBs should be initiated at low doses and titrated judiciously in order to prevent such adverse effects as hypotension and renal insufficiency. Doses should be titrated, as tolerated, to those attained in the previously mentioned trials (see Table 7.1). Monitoring and management of patients receiving ARBs should be analogous to that of ACEIs.

ALDOSTERONE ANTAGONISTS

Aldosterone antagonists are yet another class of agents available to target the RAAS. Sodium and water retention, hypokalemia, fibrosis, and ventricular remodeling are all consequences of excess aldosterone. The favorable effects of aldosterone antagonism in HF are due primarily to the inhibition of collagen deposition and fibrosis, therefore preventing ventricular remodeling.

Spironolactone was the first aldosterone antagonist studied in the HF population. The RALES trial, which compared spironolactone to placebo, was halted early after a 30% relative risk reduction in the primary endpoint of all-cause mortality was discovered during an interim analysis.[11] Eplerenone, a selective aldosterone receptor antagonist, was studied in patients post-myocardial infarction with left ventricular dysfunction (EF < 40%).[12] There was a significant reduction in mortality, risk of hospitalization due to HF, and sudden death due to cardiac causes. Unlike in the RALES trial, there were more cases of hyperkalemia and no difference in gynecomastia in the eplerenone group.

Aldosterone inhibitors are indicated in patients with symptomatic structural heart disease or those with left ventricular dysfunction after myocardial infarction (see Figure 7.1).[1] These agents are not suitable for all patients. Patients should be carefully selected and monitored closely to prevent life-threatening hyperkalemia. These agents should be avoided if serum potassium exceeds 5.5 mEq/L and if CrCl is below 30 mL/min. Eplerenone must also be avoided if patients are receiving potent CYP450 3A4 inhibitors since it is a substrate of this system. Each agent should be dosed as they were in the previously mentioned clinical trials (see Table 7.1). Initial doses should be reduced in those at risk of developing hyperkalemia.

Hyperkalemia is a risk in patients receiving an aldosterone antagonist, particularly in the elderly, those with renal dysfunction (SCr > 1.6 mg/dL), and baseline serum potassium greater than 5 mEq/L. Concurrent use with other agents such as ACEIs, ARBs, and NSAIDs may increase the risk of hyperkalemia. Renal function and serum potassium should be monitored at baseline and routinely thereafter, especially following adjustment of other medications (e.g., ACEI, ARB, diuretics).

VASODILATORS (HYDRALAZINE AND ISDN)
Isosorbide dinitrate is a venodilator commonly paired with hydralazine which is largely an arterial smooth muscle vasodilator. The combination provides a reduction in preload and afterload, leading to an improvement in SVR and cardiac output. There is some evidence to suggest that the use of hydralazine with ISDN may attenuate the nitrate tolerance frequently seen with nitrate administration.

Hydralazine and ISDN were compared to enalapril which demonstrated that the ACEI was superior in reducing mortality but hydralazine and ISDN led to a greater improvement in exercise capacity.[13] A more recent trial comparing hydralazine and ISDN to placebo in African-American patients, receiving standard therapy with ACEI and beta blockers, was published.[14] The trial was terminated early due to a significantly higher mortality observed in the placebo group. Unfortunately, 50% of patients reported headache and 30% complained of dizziness among those receiving the active treatment.

Based on these published data, ACEI are considered standard of care rather than hydralazine and ISDN. Due to lack of published data, hydralazine and ISDN should not be substituted in patients who are tolerating ACEI or who are ACEI naïve. This combination may be beneficial in those who have proven intolerance to ACEI or ARB. The use of hydralazine and ISDN is also limited by patient compliance since each drug must be administered 3–4 times daily. A high likelihood of adverse effects, such as headache and gastrointestinal complaints, can also limit patient compliance.

DIGOXIN
Digoxin has been used clinically for over 200 years. In the early twentieth century, it was demonstrated that digoxin exhibited positive inotropic effects. Decades later, the DIG trial randomized

patients with symptomatic HF and an EF < 45% to either digoxin or placebo.[15] Digoxin had no effect on all-cause mortality
compared to placebo. There was a small reduction in hospitalizations and fewer hospitalizations for worsening HF in the digoxin
group. This was the first trial involving a positive inotrope which
did not result in an increase in mortality. Two studies performed
investigated the effect of digoxin withdrawal in patients with or
without concurrent ACEI therapy.[16,17] Patients in whom digoxin
was withdrawn exhibited worsening HF symptoms and declining
exercise tolerance. Patients also exhibited a functional decline and
a decline in quality of life scores.

These studies helped establish the role of digoxin in the current treatment of HF. Digoxin should be considered in patients
with symptomatic HF and structural heart disease who are already
receiving ACEI, beta blockers, and diuretics and are persistently
symptomatic.[1] Digoxin therapy may be considered earlier in
patients with supraventricular tachyarrhythmias, such as atrial
fibrillation, if beta blockers have already been instituted. Higher
digoxin serum concentrations are no longer recommended in this
population due to the risk of toxicity. Published data suggests that
it is prudent to aim for serum digoxin concentrations of 0.5–1 ng/
mL.[18–20]

Digoxin exerts positive inotropic effects by binding to and
inhibiting Na+, K+ ATPase. Inhibition leads to a larger contractile force with each action potential. In addition to the inotropic
effects, digoxin blunts the effects of the hyperactive sympathetic
nervous system in HF patients. This is achieved by improving
baroreceptor function through inhibiting Na+, K+ ATPase in the
parasympathetic nervous system.

Digoxin is typically introduced at daily doses of 0.125–0.25 mg.
A dosage reduction may be necessary in those with renal dysfunction, the elderly, and patients with low lean body mass as digoxin
does not appreciably distribute into adipose tissue. Digoxin should
be avoided in patients with atrioventricular block without a pacemaker.

Numerous drug interactions exist with digoxin therapy.
Medications such as amiodarone, clarithromycin, erythromycin,
and verapamil can dramatically increase serum digoxin concentrations necessitating a dosage reduction. Concomitant therapy with
these agents should be done with extreme caution to reduce the
risk of digoxin toxicity.

Digoxin toxicity can manifest as cardiac, central nervous
system, and gastrointestinal effects among others. Toxicity can
result in a broad range of cardiac rhythm disturbances, including

ventricular arrhythmias, atrioventricular block, atrial arrhythmias, sinus bradycardia, and junctional tachycardia. Noncardiac effects include nausea, vomiting, visual disturbances, fatigue, dizziness, and confusion. Serum digoxin levels do not have to exceed 2 ng/ml for these effects to occur. Reversal with digoxin immune Fab should be considered in patients experiencing life-threatening side effects.

DIURETICS

Diuretics are key ingredients in the successful management of HF patients. They are often necessary to combat the water and sodium retention elicited by angiotensin II and aldosterone. Diuretics allow for a rapid improvement in signs and symptoms of HF, such as peripheral edema, pulmonary congestion, and jugular venous pressure. These agents are often used long term to maintain symptomatic relief and improve exercise compliance. Although there have not been any clinical trials evaluating the effect of diuretics on mortality, they are indicated in all patients exhibiting signs and symptoms of volume overload.[19] Diuretics should never be used alone to treat symptomatic HF. They should be used in combination with an ACEI and beta blocker to prevent further decompensation.

Diuretics, including loop and thiazide, prevent renal tubule absorption of sodium and water. Loop diuretics inhibit reabsorption of sodium in the ascending limb of the Loop of Henle, while thiazide diuretics act in the distal convoluted tubule. Bumetanide, furosemide, and torsemide, all loop diuretics, increase sodium excretion by 20–25% whereas hydrochlorothiazide and metolazone increase excretion by only 10–15%. It should also be noted that loop diuretics maintain efficacy in renal dysfunction while thiazides are less effective in patients with a creatinine clearance below 50 mL/min. Loop diuretics are, therefore, the most commonly used diuretics in the management of HF.

The goals of diuretic therapy are to improve symptoms and to achieve euvolemia. A dry weight should be targeted at which symptoms are minimized and a fluid and sodium balance has been attained. Body weights should be recorded daily to monitor for fluid retention. Patients should be advised to consult their healthcare provider if they experience a 2–3 kg weight gain over a period of 1 week.

A ceiling effect may occur with loop diuretic therapy in which there is no longer a dose response (see Table 7.2). Additional diuresis may be achieved by more frequent dosing when this occurs. Thiazide diuretics may be administered in combination with loop

TABLE 7.2. Diuretics used in the treatment of heart failure

-	Initial daily dose	Maximum daily dose
Loop diuretics		
Bumetanide	0.5–1 mg daily	10 mg daily
Furosemide	20–40 mg 1–2 times daily	600 mg/day
Torsemide	10–20 mg daily	200 mg daily
Thiazide diuretics		
Chlorothiazide	250–500 mg 1–2 times daily	1,000 mg/day
Chlorthalidone	12.5–25 mg daily	100 mg daily
Hydrochlorothiazide	25 mg 1–2 times daily	100 mg daily
Metolazone	2.5 mg daily	20 mg/day

diuretics for a synergistic effect. Diuretic therapy requires careful management. Overdiuresis can lead to hypotension, azotemia, and metabolic disturbances. Serum potassium and magnesium should be monitored. Agents such as ACEI, ARB, aldosterone antagonists, and potassium supplements may help limit hypokalemia. Diuretics may potentially worsen glomerular filtration, therefore renal function should be monitored closely.

Diuretic resistance can be attributed to medication noncompliance, dietary indiscretion, drug interactions, and malabsorption of the diuretic. Medication noncompliance is a common reason for treatment failure in this population. Patients should be counseled on the significance of compliance and the consequences of noncompliance with all of their HF medications. Excessive dietary sodium intake can blunt the diuretic effect and lead to fluid retention. Medications, such as NSAIDs, are known to attenuate the benefits of diuretics. Intravenous diuretic administration may be necessary if bowel edema is limiting absorption of oral products.

CONCLUSIONS
In summary, many efficacious pharmacological interventions are available for the treatment of heart failure as outlined above. Careful analysis of the patient and adherence to guidelines can indeed prove substantially beneficial. Several questions remain that should be answered by future studies, such as how to identify patients at greatest risk, how to cost effectively prevent sudden death, how to identify the best candidates for mechanical circulatory support devices, and how best to treat heart failure patients with preserved systolic function (diastolic heart failure) among

many others. However, a clinician's most intensive efforts should continue to focus on prevention of the heart failure epidemic, including control of hypertension and other vascular risk factors as well as lifestyle modification to eliminate known risk factors.

References

1. Hunt SA, Abraham WT, Chin MH, Feldman AM, Francis GS, Ganiats TG, Jessup M, Konstam MA, Mancini DM, Michl K, Oates JA, Rahko PS, Silver MA, Stevenson LW, Yancy CW. ACC/AHA 2005 guideline update for the diagnosis and management of chronic heart failure in the adult: a report of the American College of Cardiology/American Heart Association Task Force on Practice Guidelines (Writing Committee to Update the 2001 Guidelines for the Evaluation and Management of Heart Failure). American College of Cardiology Web Site. Available at: http://www.acc.org/clinical/guidelines/failure//index.pdf.
2. CIBIS-II Investigators and Committees (1999) The cardiac insufficiency bisoprolol study II (CIBIS-II): a randomised trial. Lancet 353:9–13.
3. Packer M, Coats AJS, Fowler MB, et al. (2001) Effect of carvedolol on survival in severe chronic heart failure. N Engl J Med 344:1651–1658.
4. MERIT-HF Study Group (1999) Effect of metoprolol CR/XL in chronic heart failure: Metoprolol CR/XL randomised intervention trial in congestive heart failure (MERIT-HF). Lancet 353:2001–2007.
5. The SOLVD investigators (1991) Effect of enalapril on survival in patients with reduced left ventricular ejection fractions and congestive heart failure. N Engl J Med 325:293–302.
6. Cicardi M, Zingale L, Bergamaschini L, Agostoni A (2004) Angioedema associated angiotensin-converting enzyme inhibitor use. Arch Intern Med 164:910–913.
7. Pitt B, Poole-Wilson PA, Segal R, et al. (2000) Effect of losartan compared with captopril on mortality in patients with symptomatic heart failure: randomised trial-the losartan heart failure survival study ELITE II. Lancet 355:1582–1587.
8. Cohn JN, Tognoni G, et al. (2001) A randomized trial of the angiotensin-receptor blocker valsartan in heart failure. N Engl J Med 345:1667–1675.
9. Pfeffer MA, Swedberg K, Granger CB, et al. (2003) Effects of candesartan on mortality and morbidity in patients with chronic heart failure: the CHARM-overall programme. Lancet 362:759–766.
10. Pfeffer MA, McMurray J, Velazquez EJ, et al. (2003) Valsartan, captopril, or both in myocardial infarction complicated by heart failure, left ventricular dysfunction, or both. N Engl J Med 349:1893–1906.
11. Pitt B, Zannad F, Remme W, et al. (1999) The effect of spironolactone on morbidity and mortality in patient with severe heart failure. N Engl J Med 341:709–717.
12. Pitt B, Remme W, Zannad F, et al. (2003) Eplerenone, a selective aldosterone blocker, in patients with left ventricular dysfunction after myocardial infarction. N Engl J Med 348:1309–1321.

13. Cohn JN, Johnson G, Zeische S, et al. (1991) A comparison of enalapril with hydralazine-isosorbide dinitrate in the treatment of chronic congestive heart failure. N Eng J Med 325:303–310.

14. Taylor AL, Ziesche S, Yancy C, et al. (2004) Combination of isosorbide dinitrate and hydralazine in blacks with heart failure. N Engl J Med 351:2049–2057.

15. The Digitalis Investigation Group (1997) The effect of digoxin on mortality and morbidity in patients with heart failure. N Engl J Med 336:525–533.

16. Packer M, Gheorghiade M, Young JB, et al. (1993) Withdrawal of digoxin from patients with chronic heart failure treated with angiotensin-converting-enzyme inhibitors. N Engl J Med 329:1–7.

17. Uretsky BF, Young JB, Shahidi FE, et al. (1993) Randomized study assessing the effect of digoxin withdrawal in patients with mild to moderate chronic congestive heart failure: results of the PROVED trial. J Am Coll Cardiol 22(4):955–962.

18. Slatton ML, Irani WN, Hall SA, et al. (1997) Does digoxin provide additional hemodynamic and autonomic benefit at higher doses in patients with mild to moderate heart failure and normal sinus rhythm? J Am Coll Cardiol 29:1206–1213.

19. Adams KF, Gheorghiaed M, Uretsky BF, et al. (2002) Clinical benefits of low serum digoxin concentrations in heart failure. J Am Coll Cardiol 39:946–953.

20. Rathore SS, Curtis JP, Wang Y, et al. (2003) Association of serum digoxin concentration and outcomes in patients with heart failure. J Am Med Assoc 289:871–878.

Chapter 8
Surgical Options in the Treatment of Heart Failure

James J. Gangemi and George L. Hicks

Heart failure continues to increase in the United States at epidemic proportions. Over 1 million myocardial infarctions occur in this country yearly, and although the mortality rate has decreased by 24%, approximately 250,000 people die before reaching the hospital. Approximately 30,000 patients each year develop congestive heart failure (CHF) with a mortality rate of 30–50% within three years. The complications of acute (ischemia, infections, or dissections) and chronic (left ventricular remodeling, valvular disease, or CHF) cardiac insults represents some of the most challenging surgical decisions and treatment. Evolving surgical therapies continue to play an increasingly important role in this rapid expanding group of patients presenting with acute or chronic heart failure.

This chapter will outline a number of surgical treatment modalities aimed at the preservation or improvement of left ventricular function. New techniques involved with acute left ventricular failure, ischemic mitral valve insufficiency, left ventricular restoration use of restraint devices, percutaneous valve implantation, apical-aortic conduits, treatment of right ventricular dysfunction, and the potential of myocardial cellular regeneration will be emphasized. The gold standard of cardiac transplantation and the emerging area of ventricular assist device will be covered in another part of this manual.

J.D. Bisognano et al. (eds.), *Manual of Heart Failure Management,*
DOI: 10.1007/978-1-84882-185-9_8, © Springer-Verlag London Limited 2009

ACUTE LEFT VENTRICULAR FAILURE

Cardiogenic Shock Associated with Myocardial Infarction

Heart failure is defined as the inability of the heart to meet the metabolic needs of the body. Cardiogenic shock is an acute state of end-organ hypoperfusion characterized by well-defined clinical parameters. Hemodynamic indices include: cardiac index <1.8 L/min/m^2, stroke index <20 mL/m^2. pulmonary capillary wedge pressure >18 mmHg, tachycardia and systemic vascular resistance >2,400 dyn-sec/cm^5. These declines in hemodynamic parameters are characterized clinically with oliguria, dyspnea, hypotension in the face of vasoconstriction and obtundation.

Because coronary occlusion is the most common cause of this lethal scenario and autopsy studies have confirmed that cardiogenic shock is the result of losing greater than 40% of left ventricular muscle, rapid coronary revascularization allowing reperfusion and infarct size reduction is the modern day credo for patients experiencing acute myocardial infarctions. Interestingly, even patients having successful revascularization of the culprit lesion can remain in or develop cardiogenic shock as reperfusion of the ischemic area of myocardium frequently results in myocardial stunning. The combination of calcium overload, free radical generation, and dysfunction of the sarcoplasmic reticulum results in impairment of myocardial function in the face of normal blood flow. It is unclear whether the delays in presentation, treatment itself, or extent of coronary disease has an impact on this phenomenon. Any of the revascularization options for acute myocardial infarction (thrombolytic agents, angioplasty, and coronary artery bypass surgery) can result in stunning, and if the remaining myocardium is incapable of supporting the metabolic needs of the body, further medical or surgical treatment is necessary. The treatment of non-transmural infarctions by either delayed PTCA or bypass surgery results in the lowest mortality as mortality for the nontransmural group peaks within 6 h of onset and decreases markedly thereafter (Figure 8.1).

In contrast the modern day treatment of acute transmural myocardial infarction necessitates 24/7 readiness of catheterization laboratories and personnel with specialized emergency room protocols available for the rapid and efficient diagnosis and treatment of patients with chest pain and clinical evidence of shock. The GISSI I and II trials demonstrated no benefit from intravenous thrombolysis in this group (mortality 70%) whereas PTCA within 6 h improved survival by 40–60%. The SHOCK trial and other studies gives further support to immediate revascularization as either PTCA or coronary artery bypass surgery within

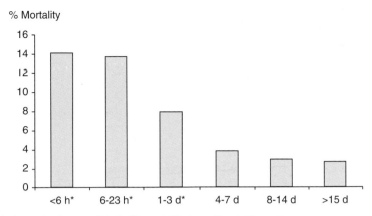

* Independently associated with mortality in multivariable analyses.

FIGURE 8.1. Hospital mortality vs. timing of CABG after transmural MI. Among patients who underwent CABG after transmural MI in New York State, mortality was more than doubled that of the baseline value when surgery was performed within 3 days of transmural MI.

TABLE 8.1. Postoperative procedures and complications

		MTI ($n = 33$)		STI ($n = 18$)		
		No.	%	No.	%	P value
IABP	3		9.1	2	11.1	>0.999
Atrial fibrillation		8	24.2	4	22.2	>0.999
Ventricular tachycardia		3	9.1	1	5.6	>0.999
Junctional rhythm		1	3.0	0	0	>0.999
Pacemaker		2	6.1	0	0	0.53
Bleeding necessitating reoperation		1	3.0	0	0	>0.999
Transfusion		7	21.2	0	0	0.04
Deep vein thrombosis		5	15.2	2	11.1	>0.999
Stroke		3	9.1	1	5.6	>0.999
Infection						
Sternal infection		2	6.6	1	5.6	>0.999
Pneumonia		5	15.2	1	5.6	0.41
Urinary tract infection		4	12.1	1	5.6	0.64
Sepsis		3	9.1	1	5.6	>0.999
Additional surgery						
Débridement		2	6.6	1	5.6	>0.999
LVAD placement		3	9.1	1	5.6	>0.999
Defibrillator implantation		2	6.1	2	11.1	0.61

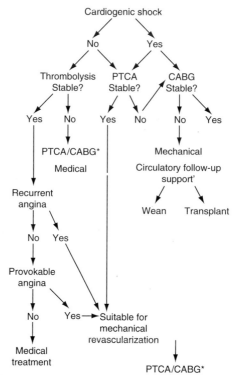

*PTCA - percutaneous transluminal coronary angioplasty: CABG -
coronary artery bypass grafting. Choice of therapy is made bassed on the
lesion(s) and comorbid factors.

*Choice of mechanical support is based on many factors (see text, along
with other chapters).

FIGURE 8.2. Acute myocardial infarction algorithm.

6 h of infarction improved one year survival. This study further
revealed that the patients <75 years of age seemed to benefit most
from this strategy. An algorithm for the decision pathways regarding acute myocardial infarction and shock as described by George
and Oz is included (Figure 8.2).

Patient support after revascularization depends on the level
of cardiac function. Although inotropes and intra-aortic balloon
support can be important, continued evidence of cardiogenic
shock despite adequate medical therapy requires the prudent but
rapid utilization of ventricular assist devices. This clinical scenario
frequently requires transportation of the patient to a center that

specializes is such technology as well as cardiac transplantation. The decision-making for the support of these patients is not always easy and some factors for consideration are listed below:

1. Is the patient a transplant candidate?
2. What is the neurologic status?
3. Cause of the cardiac dysfunction
4. Chance for return of cardiac function
5. Patient's age and size
6. Ability to anticoagulate
7. Presence of infection
8. Extent of multi-organ failure
9. The need for right and/or left ventricular support
10. The need for temporary vs. permanent ventricular assist

Ventricular assist devices will be fully covered in Chapter (9) as the differences in function, type, size, and temporary vs. permanent nature of the devices are beyond the scope of this chapter. However, ventricular assist devices used in selected patients can reverse the problems of organ damage caused by high level of inotropes, restore normal systemic circulation, and improve patient survival as noted in several recent studies. These patients may go on to cardiac transplantation, explantation of the device or destination therapy with excellent long-term outlooks. An algorithm for some decisions made regarding assist devices follows (Figure 8.3).

Surgical Treatment of Left Ventricular Remodeling
The prevalence of congestive heart failure in the United States is approximately 5 million patients, and it is increasing yearly. Ischemic cardiomyopathy is the cause of CHF in 3 million of these patients. Approximately 35–50% of patients with CHF will die within 2 years without treatment. Although medical treatments are effective in the short term, cardiac transplantation is widely accepted as the criterion standard therapy for the treatment of CHF. Unfortunately, transplantation is limited by lack of donors, is expensive, and carries many exclusions that remove it as an option for most patients. Thus, alternatives are needed for patients with advanced CHF.

The changes that occur in left ventricular geometry after myocardial infarction are termed left ventricular remodeling as the contractile units of the affected region have impaired or no function causing regional dilatation. This geometric alteration changes the normally conical left ventricle to become more globular, increasing left ventricular end systolic and diastolic volume,

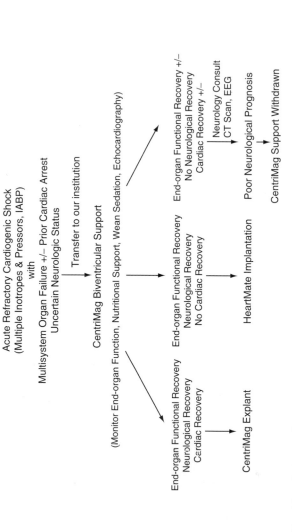

FIGURE 8.3. Algorithm depicting the management of patients transferred from outside institutions with refractory acute cardiogenic shock with MSOF. IABP, Intraaortic balloon pump; CT, computed tomography; EEG, electroencephalogram.

increasing tension on functional papillary muscles as well as increasing wall tension.

With the development of LV remodeling, progressive dimensional changes of the left ventricle can result in:

1. Decrease in LV ejection fraction
2. Progressive increase in LV end-diastolic pressure
3. Dilated cardiomyopathy with CHF
4. Mitral valve insufficiency caused by tethering of the leaflets

Indications for left ventricular restoration:

1. Anteroseptal infarction and dilated LV (end-diastolic volume index >100 mL/m^2
2. Ejection fraction <30%
3. LV regional asynergy, either dyskinesia or akinesia >35% of LV
4. Symptoms of angina, heart failure, and arrhythmias
5. Inducible ischemia on provocative testing in asymptomatic patients

Contraindications:

1. Systolic pulmonary hypertensive not associated with mitral insufficiency
2. Right ventricular dysfunction measured by RV work index
3. Regional asynergy without LV dilatation

The surgical approach for left ventricular remodeling is predicated on the concept of restoring the geometry of the left ventricle to a conical shape. As shown below the left ventricle is opened in the area of dilatation or scar and direct inspection of the interior of the LV allows the surgeon to determine the beginning area of normal myocardium. This demarcation zone is used to fashion a new LV apex utilizing a constricting stitch and apical patch. The volume of the LV is determined by the patient's preoperative LV dimensions and body surface area using a balloon template of known volume to adequately but not overly downsize the LV. Additional areas of thinning or dilatation can be plicated and the remaining LV scar is then closed to complete the repair (Figure 8.4).

The operative mortality of the Dor procedure depends upon the selection of patients excluding those with biventricular dysfunction or global left ventricular function which would preclude adequate postoperative cardiac output. The mortality rate for these procedures 3–13% which reflects the spectrum of patients

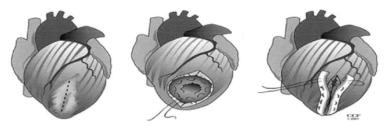

FIGURE 8.4. Surgical approach for left ventricular remodeling.

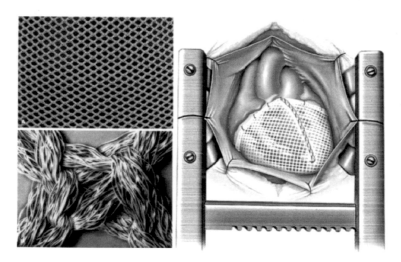

FIGURE 8.5. Cardiac support device (CSD) structure (next to the left 2 pictures). The CSD is a polyester knit construction with compliance characteristics designed to encourage beneficial reverse remodeling in dilated cardiomyopathy: (a) Photograph of an isolated area of open-weave construction (original magnification approximately ×2.5); (b) Scanning electron microscopy photograph showing node (knot; original magnification approximately ×70).(under the Left picture) Positioning and securing the CSD. The CSD hemline is attached near the atrioventricular groove through a series of interrupted sutures, starting with the posterior aspect. An anterior seam is used to create the proper device fit.

chosen for surgery, need for additional procedures and the addition of patients with significant mitral insufficiency, which will be discussed later. Improved long-term survival has been seen in patients with LVEF >20%, absence of post-op CHF and ventricular arrhythmias and control of hypertension (Table 8.1).

Left Ventricular Restraint

As demonstrated by the left ventricular restoration techniques, the preservation of conical shape or prevention of left ventricular remodeling has a positive effect on long-term LV function. To prevent left remodeling and its negative sequelae, the CorCap cardiac support device was developed through extensive animal research and now in clinical trials.

The restraint device is a fabric mesh that is surgically placed circumferentially around the heart using basilar measurements and ECHO dimensions to guide the size of restraint to be used. As shown below, the device creates a conical shape and actively resists LV geometric changes, thereby reduces LV wall stress, and LV volumes (Figure 8.5).

The Acorn clinical trial tested the safety and efficacy of LV restraint using the CorCap device. Randomized as shown below clinical and dimensional outcomes were measured (Figures 8.6 and 8.7).

The principal finding from this three year follow-up study of echocardiograms from patients enrolled in the Acorn Randomized Trial is that implantation of the CorCap Cardiac Support Device is

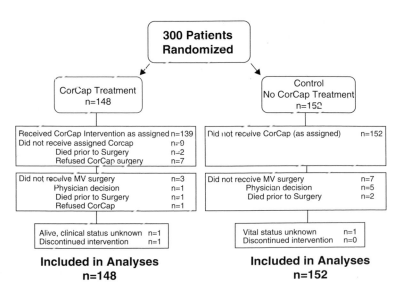

FIGURE 8.6. Randomization, treatment, and vital status of patients in the Acorn trial. (CorCap [Acorn Cardiovascular]; MV = mitral valve) (view within article).

safe in patients with heart failure and leads to beneficial cardiac remodeling that is characterized by reduced LV volume and a more elliptical LV shape. These data also suggest that the beneficial changes reported previously were durable and maintained throughout the three year follow-up period. It is also noted that the most improved outcomes were in the mitral valve repair group, reinforcing the concept that geometric stability, lack of progression of mitral insufficiency and stable LV ejection fraction improve long-term survival. These findings provide important new

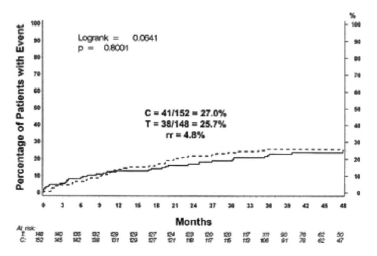

FIGURE 8.7. (under the 1 slide on the left) Mortality: June 2006. Kaplan-Meier mortality curves for the CorCap cardiac support device (CSD: Acorn Cardiovascular) treatment group (*solid line*) and the control group (*dotted line*) for patients followed out to four years. The CorCap CSD treatment.group had a lower crude mortality rate (25.7%) when compared with the control group (27.0%, risk reduction of 4.8%) but this difference was not significant. (*dotted line* = control [C]; *straight line* = treatment [T; cardiac support device].) (under the 2 slides on the right) Changes in left ventricular end-diastolic volume (LVEDV) in the two strata. In the mitral valve replacement (MVR) stratum (top), the control group (MVR surgery alone) demonstrated a progressive reduction in LVEDV. The treatment group (MVR surgery plus CorCap cardiac support device [CSD; Acorn Cardiovascular) show incremental benefit (average difference = 16.0 mL; *p* = 0.032). In the no-MVR stratum (*bottom*), the control group (medical therapy alone) shows no consistent change in LVEDV until an apparent increase during late follow-up. The treatment group (CorCap CSD) shows consistently smaller LV size (average treatment effect = 24.7 mL; *p* = 0.042).

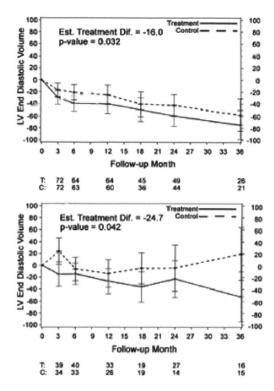

FIGURE 8.7. (continued)

information that addresses the long-term efficacy of the CorCap Cardiac Support Device. Further, there were no safety concerns with the device at three years and no clinically significant device-related complications.

More recent data in acute left remodeling suggests that used earlier in MI restraint devices may be beneficial.

Ischemic Mitral Valve Insufficiency

Mitral valve insufficiency caused by complications of myocardial ischemia or infarction is a known risk factor for long-term survival. As shown below the presence of 3–4+ mitral insufficiency had a significantly lower five-year survival when compared with similar patients having only 1–2+MR.

The treatment of significant mitral insufficiency is essential if the continued volume forces on an already compromised left ventricle are to be normalized and long-term survival improved.

Bolling, Adams, and McCarthy have all reported the effectiveness of mitral valve repair and/or replacement in this high-risk patient cohort with reduced left ventricular function.

The etiology of ischemic mitral insufficiency mirrors that of LV remodeling with globular LV changes, decreased papillary muscle function secondary to scarring, displacement and distortion of the bases of the papillary muscles, leading to valve leaflet tethering and insufficiency. Thus ischemic MR is thought to be a problem of ventricular origin as opposed to the valve itself as demonstrated below.

The surgical treatment of ischemic MR is determined by the mechanisms associated with the valve regurgitation and can include:

1. Valve annuloplasty with an undersized rigid ring
2. Annuloplasty with a deformed ring to depress the tethered segment improving coaptation
3. Restoration of normal papillary muscle tension
4. Restoring LV dimensions including distance between papillary muscles
5. Mitral valve replacement (Figure 8.8)

The use of a rigid ring is felt important due to the continued forces on the anterior and posterior annulus to continue dilation and eventual progressive valvular insufficiency.

The procedural mortality and survival follows closely the residual LV function and absence of residual mitral insufficiency in follow-up. In a study by Callifiore, 5 of 29 patients died, for a 17% actual mortality in the mitral valve repair group, versus 6 of 20 deaths, or a 30% actual mortality in the mitral valve replacement group; a significantly higher actual mortality in the mitral valve

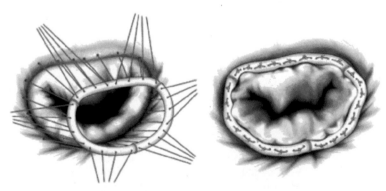

FIGURE 8.8. Mitral valve annuloplasty.

replacement group versus mitral valve repair. In regards to the actuarial survival, mitral valve repair was 83% vs. 70% for mitral valve replacement, and improvement of New York Heart Class Association at 5 years was 76% in patients undergoing mitral valve repair compared with 65% after mitral valve replacement.

Acute Mitral Valve Insufficiency

Papillary Muscle Rupture

Papillary muscle ruptured causes rapid cardiac decompensation and cardiogenic shock. After diagnosis by echocardiography and coronary angiography, an intra-aortic balloon pump is placed and emergency surgery is performed. When patients with papillary muscle infarction and elongation without rupture develop 3+ or 4+MR and congestive symptoms, surgery is indicated (Figure 8.9).

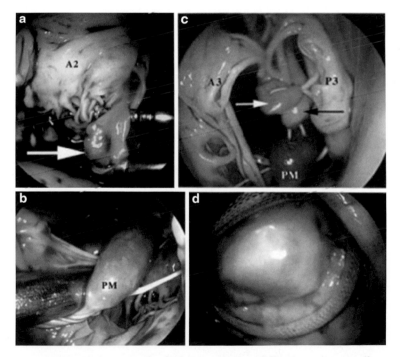

FIGURE 8.9. Restoration of valvular competence following acute papillary muscle rupture can include papillary muscle reimplantation into unaffected papillary muscle, left ventricular free wall or the existing head of the papillary muscle. A concomitant annuloplasty often performed.

Restoration of valvular competence for acute rupture can include papillary muscle reimplantation into unaffected papillary muscle, left ventricular free wall or existing head of papillary muscle. A concomitant annuloplasty to the coaptation zone is often performed. In extremely ill patients, a mitral valve replacement preserving existing chordal support is frequently the procedure of choice. Because these patients often will have only focal ventricular involvement, successful surgery without residual mitral insufficiency has better long-term survival than ischemic mitral disease and severe LV dysfunction.

Cellular Therapy for Left Ventricular Injury

Left ventricular failure secondary to myocardial cell dysfunction remains the pressing problem for the future and despite the utilization of surgical techniques and devices carries a significant long-term mortality. The future treatment of left ventricular failure may in large part reside in the new technologies surrounding the use of precursor cells growing in areas of myocardial scar or cellular dysfunction providing eventual improvement in left ventricular function. The use of stem cells, myoblasts, and skeletal muscle among others are currently under investigation utilizing tissue engineering by seeding cells in three-dimensional matrices of biodegradable polymers without artificial scaffolds to form new myocardial constructs. This technology of cell growth and cell implantation via vectors is well established but many questions are present and hopefully future answers will open this Pandora's Box allowing successful treatment of end-stage heart failure. Some of the issues to be resolved:

1. What precursor cell type provides the optimal growth, signaling, and function to improve overall ventricular function?
2. What is the optimal route of delivery?
3. What is the necessary cellular dose for initial establishment of the cell line?
4. What vectors or growth factors are critical to the process?
5. How early in the ischemic or infarction process can this therapy be successful?

Management of High Risk Patients with Aortic Stenosis

High risk patients with critical aortic stenosis are characterized by age >80, porcelain or egg shell aorta, previous coronary bypass surgery with patent grafts, severely reduced left ventricular function, or previous mediastinal infection. Conventional valve replacement in these patients carries in many cases an increased morbidity and mortality. New techniques are being evaluated for the treatment of some of these patients including apico-aortic conduits and clinical trials with percutaneous aortic valve implantation.

One of the largest series of apico-aortic conduits in elderly high risk patients has been reported by Dr John Brown in which 45 elderly patients received valved conduits for risk factors mentioned above. The procedure as pictured below is carried through a left thoracotomy and be accomplished without cardiopulmonary bypass in many cases. The operative mortality was low and mid-term durability of the prostheses was good allowing the conclusion that high risk elderly patients with no other option could be successfully palliated.

Initially carried out for compassionate use for extremely high risk patients, clinical trials are currently under way in the US and Europe to evaluate the percutaneous or apical implantation of an expandable aortic valve prosthesis. In view of the results of percutaneous AVR, the optimism expressed is premature. In fact, the only published series (6 patients affected by end-stage aortic stenosis), presented by Cribier and associates, evidenced some major drawbacks, such as perivalvular leakage, which is caused by the persistence of empty space between the percutaneous and native valves owing to calcifications and which was observed in the majority of patients. Moreover, coronary flow obstruction provoked by the valved stent and atheroembolism of calcific debris during the positioning of the device is possible. Grube and colleagues have recently described 1 single case of implantation of self-expandable valve prosthesis by the retrograde approach, which was deemed to facilitate coaxial positioning and to reduce the risk of perivalvular leakage, but required extracorporeal circulatory support (ECC) as a "safety measure." In fact, some intraprocedural complications, such as ejection of the valve into the ascending aorta at the time of balloon inflation or hemodynamic collapse after balloon predilation, have been reported. Finally, several technical difficulties have been described for both the antegrade and retrograde approach, so that a transapical access through a median sternotomy has been hypothesized. However, a percutaneous AVR that necessitates either a median sternotomy or ECC no longer sounds like percutaneous AVR. There are no approved percutaneous aortic valves in the US, and the future of this technology will depend on careful controlled evaluation of safety, durability, and outcomes in comparison to the known results with standard aortic replacement techniques or the use of apex to aortic conduits (Figure 8.10).

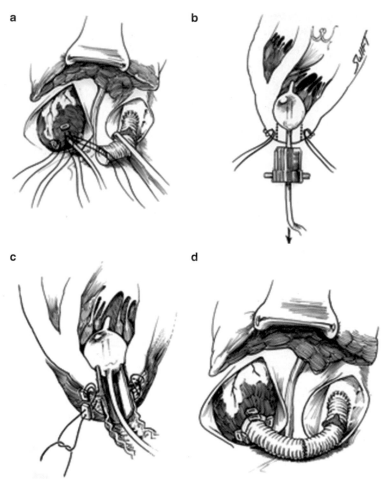

FIGURE 8.10. Placement of an apico-aortic conduit from the apex of the left ventricle to the mid-portion of the descending thoracic aorta.

Percutaneous Valve Implantation

Percutaneous heart replacement is an old initiative that has regained both enthusiasm and technological improvement from nitinol technology developed by interventional cardiologists and industry. Although there are no approved percutaneous valves in the US at the present time, trials are currently being carried out to assess efficacy, safety, and outcome. A position paper written by a combined committee of the Society of Thoracic Surgeons,

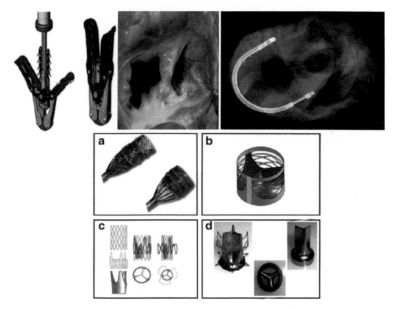

FIGURE 8.11. Examples of various percutaneous valves currently under investigation. Although an evolving technology, careful assessment of efficacy, safety, and outcome is still needed.

the American Association for Thoracic Surgery and the Society of Cardiovascular Angiography and Intervention emphasizes the need for well-designed clinical trials with success dependent upon the close collaboration of cardiology and cardiac surgery.

Multiple devices for the treatment of mitral insufficiency (Evalve and coronary sinus compression devices) and aortic stenosis (currently three devices being tested) require careful evaluation and long-term follow-up to be certain that in the zeal to treat patients with percutaneous techniques true improvement and not harm is the outcome (Figure 8.11).

Right Ventricular Failure

Although the physiology of heart failure can be applied to both the right and left ventricles, there are some causes of heart failure that are unique to the right ventricle. Right ventricular (RV) failure affects approximately 1 in 20 people. The manifestations of RV failure can include elevated jugular venous distention, hepatomegaly, ascites, peripheral edema, dyspnea on exertion, and weight gain. Conditions that cause RV failure fall under the categories of cardiac, parenchymal pulmonary disease, and pulmonary vascular disease.

Cardiac Causes
  Left systolic or diastolic dysfunction
  Coronary artery disease causing right ventricular infarction
  Valvular disease
      Pulmonary valve disease
      Tricuspid valve disease
  Constrictive pericardial disease

Parenchymal Pulmonary Disease
  Chronic obstructive pulmonary disease
  Interstitial lung disease (such as sarcoidosis)
  Adult respiratory distress syndrome (ARDS)

Pulmonary Vascular Disease
  Pulmonary embolism
  Pulmonary arterial hypertension (PAH)
      Primary PAH
      Idiopathic PAH
      Familial PAH
      Secondary to congenital heart disease, connective tissue
  disease, HIV, persistent pulmonary hypertension of the newborn

Certainly in the setting of acute RV failure, the underlying cause
needs to be addressed to the extent possible. If treatment of the
underlying etiology is unsuccessful or not possible, attempts
should be made to maximize right ventricular performance.
According to the Frank-Starling principle, volume loading may
improve RV output (even in the setting of RV contractile dysfunction). Invasive monitoring (central venous or pulmonary artery
catheters) is often necessary to determine the optimal filling pressures because excessive volume loading may be detrimental to the
RV contractile function. Inotropic support using agents such as
dobutamine or milrinone may improve RV contractile function,
especially in the setting of high pulmonary artery pressures. In few
cases when RV failure persists despite optimizing function using
the above strategies, right ventricular assist devices are required.

References
1. John R, Liao K, Lietz K, et al. Experience with the Levitronix
   CentriMag circulatory support system as a bridge to decision in
   patients with refractory acute cardiogenic shock and multisystem
   organ failure. J Thorac Cardiovasc Surg. 2007;134:351–358.
2. George I, Oz M. Myocardial Revascularization after Acute Myocardial
   Infarction. LH, Cohn Cardiac Surgery in the Adult. New York:
   McGraw-Hill, 2008:669–696.

3. Goldberg RJ, Gore JM, Alpert JS, et al. Cardiogenic shock after acute myocardial infarction. N Engl J Med 1991;325:1117.
4. Gacioch GM, Ellis SG, Lee L, et al. Cardiogenic shock complicating acute myocardial infarction: the use of coronary angioplasty and the integration of the new support devices into patient management. J Am Coll Cardiol 1992;19:647.
5. Hochman JS, Sleeper LA, Webb JG, et al. Early revascularization in acute myocardial infarction complicated by cardiogenic shock. SHOCK Investigators. Should We Emergently Revascularize Occluded Coronaries for Cardiogenic Shock. N Engl J Med 1999;341:625.
6. Hochman JS, Sleeper LA, White HD, et al. One-year survival following early revascularization for cardiogenic shock. JAMA 2001;285:190.
7. Wackers FJ, Lie KI, Becker AE, et al. Coronary artery disease in patients dying from cardiogenic shock or congestive heart failure in the setting of acute myocardial infarction. Br Heart J 1976;38:906.
8. Gutovitz AL, Sobel BE, Roberts R. Progressive nature of myocardial injury in selected patients with cardiogenic shock. Am J Cardiol 1978;41:469.
9. Rahimtoola SH. The hibernating myocardium. Am Heart J 1989;117:211.
10. Oz MC, Goldstein DJ, Pepino P, Weinberg AD, Thompson SM, Catanese KA, et al. Screening scale predicts patients successfully receiving long-term implantable left ventricular assist devices. Circulation 1995;92(suppl II):169–173.
11. Morris R, Pochettino A, O'Hara M, Gardner T, Acker MA. Emergent mechanical support in the community: improvement with early transplant referral. J Heart Lung Transplant 2005;24:764–768.
12. Samuels LE, Holmes EC, Thomas MP, Entwistle III JC, Morris RJ, Narula J, et al. Management of acute cardiac failure with mechanical assist: experience with the Abiomed BVS 5000. Ann Thorac Surg 2001;71:S67–S72.
13. Morgan JA, Stewart AS, Brian J, Oz MC, Naka Y. Role of the Abiomed BVS 5000 device for short-term support and bridge to transplantation. ASAIO J 2004;50:360–363.
14. Couper GS, Dekkers RJ, Adams DH. The logistics and cost-effectiveness of circulatory support: advantages of the Abiomed BVS 5000. Ann Thorac Surg 1999;68:646–649.
15. Pagani FD, Lynch W, Swaniker F, Dyke DB, Bartlett R, Koelling T, et al. Extracorporeal life support to left ventricular assist device bridge to heart transplant. A strategy to optimize survival and resource utilization. Circulation 1999;100:II206–II210.
16. Pagani FD, Aaronson KD, Swaniker F, Bartlett RH. The use of extra-corporeal life support in adult patients with primary cardiac failure as a bridge to implantable left ventricular assist device. Ann Thorac Surg 2001;71:77–81.
17. Smedira NG, Moazami N, Golding CM, McCarthy PM, Apperson-Hansen C, Blackstone EH, et al. Clinical experience with 202 adults receiving extracorporeal membrane oxygenation for cardiac failure: survival at 5 years. J Thorac Cardiovas Surg. 2001;122:92–102.

18. Dor V, Sabatier M, Di Donato M, Montiglio F, Toso A, Maioli M. Efficacy of endoventricular patch plasty in large postinfarction akinetic scar and severe left ventricular dysfunction: comparison with a series of large dyskinetic scars. *J* Thorac Cardiovasc Surg 1998;116:50–59.

19. Di Donato M, Sabatier M, Dor V, et al. Effects of the Dor procedure on left ventricular dimension and shape and geometric correlates of mitral regurgtitation one year after surgery. J Thorac Cardiovasc Surg 2001;121:91–96.

20. Suma H, Isomura T, Horri T, et al. Nontransplant cardiac surgery for end-stage cardiomyopathy. J Thorac Cardiovasc Surg 2000;119: 1233–1245.

21. Menicanti L, Di Donato M. The Dor procedure: What has changed after fifteen years of clinical practice? J Thorac Cardiovasc Surg 2002;124:886–890.

22. Cohn JN. Structural basis for heart failure: ventricular remodeling and its pharmacological inhibition Circulation 1995;91:2504–2507.

23. Douglas PS, Morrow R, Ioli A, Reicheck N. Left ventricular shape, afterload, and survival in idiopathic dilated cardiomyopathy J Am Coll Cardiol 1989;13:311–315.

24. Vasan RS, Larson MG, Benjamin EJ, Evans JC, Levy D. Left ventricular dilation and the risk of congestive heart failure in people without myocardial infarction N Engl J Med 1997;336:1350–1355.

25. Oz MC, Konertz WF, Kleber FX, et al. Global surgical experience with the Acorn cardiac support device J Thorac Cardiovasc Surg 2003;126:983–991.

26. Ellis SG, Whitlow PL, Raymond RE, Schneider JP. Impact of mitral regurgitation on long-term survival after percutaneous coronary intervention. Am J Cardiol 2002;89:315–318.

27. Gillinov AM, Wierup PN, Blackstone EH, Bishay ES, Cosgrove DM, White J, Lytle BW, McCarthy PM. Is repair preferable to replacement for ischemic mitral regurgitation? J Thorac Cardiovasc Surg 2001;122:1125–1141.

28. Calafiore AM, Gallina S, Di Mauro M, Gaeta F, Iaco AL, D'Alessandro S, Mazzei V, Di Giammarco G. Mitral valve procedure in dilated cardiomyopathy: repair or replacement? Ann Thorac Surg 2001; 71:1146–1153.

29. Bolling SF, Deeb GM, Brunsting LA, Bach DS. Early outcome of mitral valve reconstruction in patients with end-stage cardiomyopathy. J Thorac Cardiovasc Surg 1995;109:676–683.

30. Wollert KC, Drexler H: Clinical applications of stem cells for the heart. Circ Res 2005; 96:151.

31. Reffelmann T, Kloner RA. Cellular cardiomyoplasty - Cardiomyocytes, skeletal myoblasts, or stem cells for regenerating myocardium and treatment of heart failure? Cardiovasc Res 2003;58:358.

32. Brown JW. Management of Complex Aortic Stenosis - Role of the Apex-toAortic conduit. AATS/STS Adult Cardiac Symposium, 2006.

33. Cribier A, Eltchaninoff H, Tron C, Bauer F, Agatiello C, Sebagh L, et al. Early experience with percutaneous transcatheter implantation of heart valve prosthesis for the treatment of end-stage inoperable patients with calcific aortic stenosis. J Am Coll Cardiol 2004;43.698–703.

34. Cribier A, Eltchaninoff H, Bash A, Borenstein N, Tron C, Bauer F, et al. Percutaneous transcatheter implantation of an aortic valve prosthesis for calcific aortic stenosis. First human case description. Circulation 2002;106:3006–3008.

35. Grube E, Laborde JC, Zickman B, Gerckens U, Federhoff T, Sauren B, et al. First report on a human percutaneous transluminal implantation of a self-expanding valve prosthesis for interventional treatment of aortic valve stenosis. Catheter Cardiovasc Interv 2005;66:465–469.

36. Vassiliades TA, Block PC, Cohn LH, et al: The clinical development of percutaneous heart valve technology: A position statement of the Society of Thoracic Surgeons, American Association of Thoracic Surgery, and the Society of Cardiovascular Angiography and Intervention. J Am Coll Cardiol 2005;45:1554.

37. Cribier A, Savin T, Saoudi N, et al: Percutaneous transluminal valvuloplasty of acquired aortic stenosis in elderly patients: An alternative to valve replacement? Lancet 1986;1:63.

Chapter 9
Mechanical Circulatory Assist Devices

Dana Shannon, William Hallinan, and H. Todd Massey

OVERVIEW

Mechanical circulatory support devices (MCSDs) have gained acceptance over the past 10 years as a therapy for the treatment of heart failure. These devices can restore cardiac output, maintaining perfusion and thus supplying oxygen to the vital organs. In recent years there has been a push to develop smaller, more efficient, and durable pumps that allow patients to have a better quality of life.

The first artificial heart programs were developed in the late 1950s and early 1960s. These stemmed from the successful implementation of cardiopulmonary bypass in 1953 by Gibbon.[1] With the inception of the National Institutes of Heath (NIH) artificial heart program in 1964, there was a push in the development of clinically useful ventricular assist devices.[2] In the mid 1990s, devices began to receive approval from the Food and Drug administration (FDA) to support patients awaiting heart transplantation. The HeartMate ventricular assist system was the first FDA-approved implantable device for bridge to transplant in 1994. The NHLBI has invested over $400 million in the development of mechanical circulatory devices over the past four decades clearly realizing the need for this type of therapy.[2,3] Currently there are approximately 500,000 new heart failure patients per year in the United States with estimates of approximately 300,000 deaths per annum in the United States due to heart failure.[4] Current cardiac transplant volumes in the United States and worldwide

J.D. Bisognano et al. (eds.), *Manual of Heart Failure Management*,
DOI: 10.1007/978-1-84882-185-9_9, © Springer-Verlag London Limited 2009

have been stymied due to a lack of suitable donors with average volumes in the United States of approximately 2,200 transplants per year. The actual rate of heart transplant per million populations in the United States has decreased 14%[5] during the last decade despite an increasing rate of hospital admissions for heart failure of approximately 159% during the past decade.[6] This discrepancy between need and availability and applicability of heart transplantation to a much larger population has led to resurgence in the field of mechanical circulatory devices. The vast majority of patients with end-stage heart failure do not qualify for a heart transplant due to a multitude of factors most notable being age limitations where the incidence of heart failure approaches 10 per 1,000 in those 65 years and older.[7] The rational for the development of MCSDs was clearly evident - an unlimited resource that is readily available and can not only be applied to the small population of patients awaiting heart transplant requiring bridge therapy but also be applied to that much larger population of heart transplant ineligible patients suffering from end-stage heart failure who previously only had palliative end-of-life care available after failing conventional medical therapy.

The favorable results that were seen in the bridge-to-transplant population lead to the design of the NIH sponsored multicenter randomized evaluation of mechanical assistance for the treatment of congestive heart failure (REMATCH) trial. REMATCH evaluated the efficacy and safety of permanent/destination left ventricular assist device (LVAD) support in patients with chronic end-stage heart failure, compared to patients receiving optimal medical management. Patients were enrolled in the pilot phase in 1996 and the analysis of the multiinstitutional trial was reported in 2001. This trial from almost a decade ago found that the LVAD population doubled the 1-year survival rate, compared with optimal medial management. In addition, patients with LVADs had a highly significant improvement in their quality of life and functional status.[3] The REMATCH trial provided the evidence to support the decision of the FDA to approve the HeartMate VE for destination/lifetime therapy in 2002. The HeartMate VE was Medicare approved for permanent therapy in end-stage heart failure in 2003.[8] Today, the next generation of pumps are in clinical trials, awaiting FDA approval for both bridge-to-transplant and destination therapy.

Recently, in April of 2008, the FDA approved the use of the first of a second generation of pumps the HeartMate II LVAD as a Bridge-to-Transplant device. In a prospective, multicenter study without a concurrent control group, 133 patients with end-stage heart failure who were on a waiting list for heart transplantation underwent implantation of a continuous-flow rotary pump. The survival rate during support was 89% at 1 month, 75% at 6 months, and 68% at 12 months. Circulatory support therapy was found to be associated with a significant improvement in functional status, as accessed with a 6-min walk test, and in NYHA functional class and quality of life (according to the Minnesota Living with Heart Failure and Kansas City Cardiomyopathy questionnaires).[9] The improvement in 6-min walk test was substantial with an average improvement of 373 m in a group of patients who before implant could not walk due to the severity of their heart failure.[10]

UTILIZATION OF MECHANICAL CIRCULATORY SUPPORT DEVICES

Currently, MCSDs are broken down into distinct types of pumps based on their design as well as there indications for use. Current FDA-approved indications for pump use include bridge-to-recovery, bridge-to-transplant, and permanent lifetime therapy. The type of pumps based on design can be either paracorporeal or intracorporeal in relation to the actual location of the pump. The pumps may be either pulsatile/displacement pumps or nonpulsatile continuous flow pumps inclusive of the rotary impeller type or centrifugal type. The pumps may have bearings or be bearing-less as in the totally magnetically levitated pumps. The utilization of the different systems is determined most notably by the clinical situation and specifically the ultimate goals of therapy. A single institution may have an array of different pumps that are utilized in different clinical scenarios. At our institution we typically divide the pumps into two groups - those intended for acute decompensated support and those for more elective implant for chronic heart failure. The ultimate goal of therapy is paramount to the specific device utilized being either short-term (days to weeks) or long-term (years) support in relation to the ultimate goals of recovery, transplant, or permanent lifetime therapy.

In the acute setting, short-term support devices are utilized. The length of support is typically 7–14 days at which time the pumps are removed or the patient is transitioned to a long-term pump. These MCSDs include the Abiomed BVS 5000, Levitronix Centrimag, Impella Recover 2.5/5.0, and the TandemHeart percutaneous VAD.

In the setting of chronic heart failure, MCSDs are utilized when it is recognized that the symptoms of heart failure can no longer be managed with medical therapy alone. The devices that are used in this setting are the long-term MCSDs. Long-term devices are utilized either as bridge to heart transplant devices or as destination/permanent lifetime therapy devices. These include both the pulsatile volume-displacement devices and the newer technology implantable continuous flow-rotary impeller and centrifugal pumps. The devices in this category include the pulsatile/displacement pump HeartMate XVE as well as the second generation nonpulsatile rotary impeller pumps HeartMate II, to Ventrassist, Micromed DeBakey, and Jarvik 2000. The third generation of these devices will include pumps such as the implantable totally magnetically levitated bearing-less centrifugal pumps, Levacor and the HeartMate III.

In addition, the pumps of the future will be completely implantable systems utilizing transcutaneous energy transfer system (TETS) technology. TETS can provide power to an implanted ventricular assist device across an unbroken layer of skin. This will eliminate the necessity of the driveline utilized for powering the device and the potential infections risks associated with a percutaneous tether. Refinements in TETS technology and battery technology are currently underway and it is predicted that totally implantable systems will be available in the next few years.

Total artificial heart pumps are orthotopically implanted and the native heart ventricles are excised. The first successful utilization of temporary total artificial heart was by Denton Cooley in 1969 utilizing a device developed by Liotta and DeBakey.[11] The first permanent implant of a TAH system was done in 1982; a Jarvik-7 was implanted into Dr. Barney Clark by Dr. William DeVries at the University of Utah. Dr. Clark was supported on the Jarvik-7 for a total of 112 days.[12,13] The Syncardia Cardiowest TAH-t system was approved as a temporary system for bridging to cardiac transplant by the FDA in 2004.[14] Medicare approved reimbursement for the Syncardia Cardiowest TAH-t on 5/1/2008 reversing its 1986 noncoverage policy for total artificial heart systems.

PHYSIOLOGY OF VENTRICULAR ASSIST DEVICE USE

The goal of mechanical circulatory support is to restore normal physiologic blood flow to the body and prevent end-organ dysfunction. In doing so the ventricle is unloaded thereby decreasing the myocardial workload and reducing the myocardial oxygen demand. Use of a VAD will reduce preload, myocardial wall tension and oxygen consumption.[15] Numerous studies have highlighted the ability of MCSDs to adequately restore tissue perfusion and maintain as well as reverse end-organ dysfunction.

In the realm of cardiac recovery, one needs to be clear in the discussion in relation to acute cardiomyopathy and chronic cardiomyopathy. The success in bridging to recovery in acute cardiomyopathy is well established and has relatively high successful explant rates in acute processes such as viral cardiomyopathy, postpartum cardiomyopathy, postcardiotomy states, and primary graft dysfunction in heart transplant Utilization of mechanical support to recover the chronically failing heart has not been as successful.[16] The unloading of the ventricle in chronic heart failure with MCSDs has revealed reverse remodeling in cellular and molecular markers. Reverse remodeling has been most extensively studied in paired tissue samples obtained at the time of VAD implant and subsequently at the time of explant. In chronic heart failure, it is well documented that LVAD therapy can reverse the phenotypic expression of heart failure at a molecular and cellular level but despite this clinically relevant data successful explant and sustainable recovery only occurs in approximately 5% of chronic heart failure patients.[17] The exciting opportunity of potentially being able to support and recover myocardial function in chronic heart failure patients continues to be actively pursued in numerous ongoing clinical trials utilizing novel molecular targets, stem cell therapy, and tissue regeneration strategies.

In mechanical circulatory support and especially in the use of lifetime therapy, markers of patient functional status as well as quality of life measurements have been studied extensively. In all randomized studies involving long-term mechanical circulatory devices vs. conventional therapy, there has been significant mortality and functional benefits but even more importantly significant improvements in quality of life measurements. Exercise capacity, as measured by peak oxygen consumption, has been shown to increase significantly 2 months after LVAD implantation.[18] Circulatory support with the HeartMate II continuous-flow pump significantly improved the hemodynamic status of patients and was associated with significant improvements in functional status, as assessed with a 6-min walk, and in NYHA functional class and quality of life, as measured by both the Minnesota Living with Heart Failure and Kansas City Cardiomyopathy questionnaires.[19]

EVALUATION AND CONSIDERATION OF PATIENTS FOR MCSDS

Patients who are considered for MCSDs present in a multitude of settings and health states. Appropriate and timely patient selection is crucial to the ultimate success of mechanical circulatory support therapy. There is clearly a point in time in both acute cardiogenic shock populations and in chronic heart failure populations where implantation of these devices is futile despite restoring normal tissue perfusion. Obviously the acute shock patient will have a more rapid progression to these points of no return vs. the chronic heart failure patients who have a more insidious onset. Predictability of survival of the implant procedure has gained significant attention in the past few years as device therapy strategies have improved (Figure 9.1).

Survivals of >80% in a low-risk chronic heart failure group were reported at 1 year vs. 10% for a high-risk population in

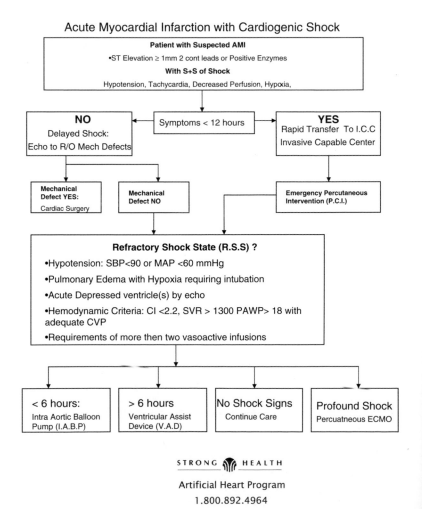

FIGURE 9.1. Acute myocardial infarction with cardiogenic shock.

the post-REMATCH era illustrating the significant differences in survival attributable to proper patient selection criteria.[20] Many of the consistent preoperative markers of poor outcomes in various studies in both acute and chronic heart failure populations include elevations in the systemic inflammatory response – WBC, temperature, CRP levels; established end-organ failure – renal, hepatic, and pulmonary: elevated total bilirubin, low urine output, elevated creatnine, requirement for mechanical ventilation. Those especially pertinent to the chronic heart failure include malnutrition/cachexia and loss of the ability of the right ventricle to perform adequate work due to longstanding overload as evidenced by reduced PAP and RVSWI.

The chronic heart failure patient population may present to the healthcare provider in either the outpatient or inpatient setting. When seen in the outpatient setting there are tools that can be used to assist the provider in the decisions surrounding MCSD patient selection (Figure 9.2).

The Office Evaluation for Heart Assist Therapy outlines several risk factors, if there is a presence of >4 factors, the patient should be evaluated for MCS. This tool can be utilized when evaluating the inpatient heart failure patient population as well. Key points that should direct a provider to look at MCSD as an option for heart failure therapy include

- Inotrope-dependent patients/Home Inotropes
- Multiple readmissions within the last 6 months for Class IIIb/IV heart failure symptoms
- Cardio-renal limitations to using ACE inhibitors/beta blockers

– Decreased systemic BP/increased creatinine
- Class III heart failure with the following indicators

– Early end-organ dysfunction
    – Hyponatremia
    – Systemic hypotension
    – Cachexia

The Contraindications for Referral for Long-Term MCSD therapy include a life expectancy of less than 2 years, related to a noncardiac condition, irreversible right heart failure, irreversible end-organ damage, significant substance abuse, and psychological barriers.

Patients who present in an acute cardiogenic shock state must be immediately assessed for MCSD candidacy. Time to support effects the outcome when looking at myocardial recovery. It is felt that mechanical circulatory support should be implemented

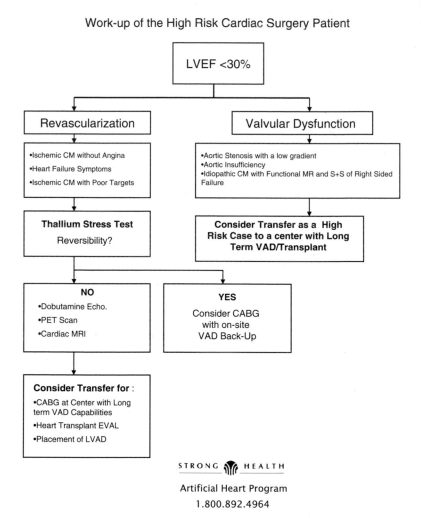

FIGURE 9.2. Work-up of the high-risk cardiac surgery patient.

within 6–12 h of the initial onset of refractory cardiogenic shock to have any meaningful hope of survival.

INTERMACS

Interagency Registry for Mechanically Assisted Circulatory Support (INTERMACS) is a registry that includes data on all dischargeable MCSDs. The goals of the registry include facilitating the refinement

TABLE 9.1. INTERMACS (interagency registry for mechanically assisted circulatory support)

PROFILE-LEVEL	Official Shorthand	General time frame for support
INTERMACS LEVEL 1	"Crash and burn"	Hours
INTERMACS LEVEL 2	"Sliding fast"	Days to week
INTERMACS LEVEL 3	Stable but Dependent	Weeks
INTERMACS LEVEL 4	"Frequent flyer"	Weeks to few months, if baseline restored
INTERMACS LEVEL 5	"Housebound"	Weeks to months
INTERMACS LEVEL 6	"Walking wounded"	Months, if nutrition and activity maintained
INTERMACS LEVEL 7	Advanced Class III	

of patient selection to maximize outcomes with current and new device options. The registry will identify predictors of good outcomes as well as risk factors for adverse events after device implantation. Providers will utilize INTERMACS to develop consensus "best practice" guidelines to improve clinical management by reducing short- and long-term complications of MCSD therapy. The data collected will guide the application and the evolution of next generation devices. Current application of INTERMACS data is utilized in determining a time frame for mechanical support through a patient stratification level (Table 9.1).

FUTURE OF MECHANICAL CIRCULATORY SUPPORT

The goal for future MCSD technology is increased utilization in the acute shock population where mortalities remain at approximately 50% with current treatment paradigms as well as increased utilization as permanent therapy in those patients with medically refractory chronic heart failure. The technology continues to evolve and current available technology offers reliable and durable results with well-documented significant mortality benefits and quality of life benefits to a range of heart failure patients. MCSD therapy has offered significant survival and quality of life benefits to end stage heart failure patients who perviously had survival similar to lung cancer and pancreatic cancer. Most importantly though are the quality of life benefits seen with MCSD therapy returning previously patients to active and enjoyable lifestyles. The future of this therapy is now as evidenced by the Joint Commissions statement that all certified destination therapy centers require all qualifying patients' access to this therapy. The field of mechanical circulatory support will continue to grow and improve as complementing technology develops.

References

1. Liotta D,Hall C, Henly W, et al. Prolonged assisted circulation during and after cardiac or aortic surgery. Am J Cardiol 1963;12:399.
2. Oz MC, Gelijns AC, Miller L, et al. Left ventricular assist devices as permanent heart failure therapy: the price of progress. Ann Surg 2003;238:577–585.
3. Cowie M, Wood D, Coats A. Incidence and aetiology of heart failure. A population – based study. Eur Heart J 1999;20:421.
4. Hunt S, et al. ACC/AHA Guidelines for the Evaluation and Management of Chronic Heart Failure in the Adult: A Report of the American College of Cardiology/American Heart Association Task Force on Practice Guidelines, 2001.
5. Mulligan MS, Shearon TH, Weill D, et al. Heart and lung transplantation in the United States, 1997–2006. Am J Transplant 2008;8(part 2):977–987.
6. American Heart Association. 2001 Heart and Stroke Statistical Update. Dallas, TX: American Heart association, 2000.
7. Jessup M, Brozena S. Medical progress heart failure. N Engl J Med 2003;348:2007–2018.
8. Frazier OH, Kirklin J Mechanical Circulatory Support. ISHLT Monograph Series, vol. 1, 2006.
9. Miller LW, Pagani FD, Russell SD, et al. Use of continuous-flow device in patients awaiting heart transplantation. N Engl J Med 2007;357(9):885–896.
10. Boyle A, Rogers J, et al. American College Cardiology 2008.
11. Cooley D, Liotta D, Hallman G. Orthotopic cardiac prothesis for two-staged cardiac replacement. Am J Cardiol 1969; 24:723.
12. DeVries W. Clinical use of the total artificial heart. N Engl J Med 1984;310:273–278.
13. DeVries W. The permanent artificial heart: four case reports. J Am Med Assoc 1988;259:849–859.
14. Frazier OH, Kirklin J. Mechanical Circulatory Support. ISHLT Monograph Series, vol. 1, 2006.
15. Scherr K, Jensen L, Koshal A. Mechanical circulatory support as a bridge to cardiac transplantation: toward the 21st century. Am J Crit Care 1999;8:324–337.
16. Mancini DM, et al. Low incidence of myocardial recovery after left ventricular assist device implantation in patients with chronic heart failure. Circulation 1998;98:2383–2389.
17. Mancini DM, et al.. Low incidence of myocardial recovery after left ventricular assist device implantation in patients with chronic heart failure. Circulation 1998;98:2383–2389.

18. Radovancevic B, Vrtovec B, Frazier OH. Left ventricular assist devices: an alternative to medical therapy for end stage heart failure. Curr Opin Cardiol 2003;18:210–214.
19. Miller, LW, Pagani, FD, Russell, SD, et al. Use of continuous-flow device in patients awaiting heart transplantation. N Engl J Med 2007;357(9).885–896.
20. Leitz K, et al. Outcomes of left ventricular assist device implantation in the post-REMATCH era: Implications for patient selection. Circulation 2007;116:497–505.

Chapter 10
Cardiac Transplantation

Grzegorz Pietrasik, Jean Huether, and Leway Chen

INTRODUCTION

The beginning of heart transplantation is dated back to the early experiments of Alexis Carrel, French surgeon, and a pioneer of vascular surgery. At the University of Chicago, in early 1900s, Carrel performed his first experimental transplant. He used canine heart and lung transplanting them onto the neck of an adult dog.[1] In the late 1920s, at the Mayo Clinic, Frank C. Mann worked on both renal and heart transplantation.[2] Mann improved surgical techniques and recognized that majority of failures of transplanted organs were due to organ rejection.[3] The first animal intrathoracic orthotropic heart transplantations were performed by Goldberg, Berman, and Akman at the University of Maryland in 1958.[4] First heart transplantation in human was performed by James Hardy at the University of Mississippi in 1964. It was xenotransplantation of primate heart (chimpanzee) to 68-year-old man bed-bound with severe coronary heart disease. Originally, it was planned to use a human heart but the patient became clinically unstable before a human heart was available. The surgical team decided to transplant chimpanzee heart. Unfortunately, the transplanted heart was too small to provide sufficient hemodynamic support and failed after 2 h.[5] The first human-to-human heart transplantation was performed by Christiaan Barnard and his team on December 3, 1967 in South Africa. The recipient was 54-year-old Louis Washkansky, a patient with severe coronary heart disease, and a donor was a 24-year-old woman who died in a car accident. Initially recipient recovered well, but died because of pneumonia

J.D. Bisognano et al. (eds.), *Manual of Heart Failure Management*,
DOI: 10.1007/978-1-84882-185-9_10, © Springer-Verlag London Limited 2009

18 days after the surgery.[6] First American human-to-human heart transplant was performed by Kantrowitz at Maimonides Hospital in Brooklyn on December 6, 1967. The recipient was a 17-day-old male baby with Ebstein anomaly who received a heart of a 2-day-old male infant with anencephaly. The recipient died within 7 h after the surgery as a result of metabolic and respiratory acidosis. Barnard performed his second heart transplantation on January 2, 1968. Patient recovered and survived next 20 months; died because of chronic rejection in August 1969. Currently, the orthotropic cardiac transplantation is the method of choice in the treatment of the end-stage heart failure. According to the 2005 report from the Registry of the International Society for Heart and Lung Transplantation (ISHLT), approximately 4,000 heart transplants are performed worldwide annually.[7] The unadjusted 1-year, 5-year, and 10-year survival rates of heart transplant graft for the cohort of the patient transplanted between the years 1982 and 2004, were approximately 85%, more than 70%, and 50%, respectively. After the initial steep in the survival during the first 6 months, the survival decreased with linear rate of approximately 3.4% per year.[8]

INDICATION AND CONTRAINDICATIONS FOR CARDIAC TRANSPLANTATION

Indications
Accepted, probable, and inadequate indications for cardiac transplantation are summarized in Table 10.1. Patients in cardiogenic shock and heart failure refractory to medical therapy, on inotropic support and/or ventricular assist device benefit the most from cardiac transplantation. For the patients with chronic heart failure the most important method of assessing benefit of cardiac transplantation is cardiopulmonary stress testing (CST).

Cardiopulmonary Stress Testing and Oxygen Consumption at Peak Exercise
CST is a class I indication for the evaluation of an exercise capacity and the response to therapy in heart failure patients considered for heart transplantation,[9] and it is recognized by the International Society for Heart and Lung Transplantation (ISHLT) as the most objective method of assessing indication and prognosis prior and after the heart transplant. CST measures patient's oxygen consumption at peak exercise (VO_2max). VO_2max below normal is most commonly caused by inability of the heart to appropriately increase cardiac output. VO_2max less than 10 mL/kg/min is associated with very poor short-term prognosis with 1-year survival

TABLE 10.1. Indications for cardiac transplant listing

Accepted indications for listing
Cardiogenic shock or low output state requiring mechanical or inotropic support
Advanced symptomatic heart failure with peak oxygen consumption (VO_2) < 10 mL/kg/min with achievement of anaerobic threshold
NYHA class IV, angina pectoris or heart failure due to advanced hypertrophic or restrictive cardiomyopathy
Refractory angina pectoris consistently limiting day-to-day activities with coronary anatomy that is not amenable to angioplasty, atherectomy, or coronary bypass grafting
Recurrent symptomatic life-threatening ventricular arrhythmias uncontrolled by all appropriate medical and surgical modalities

Probable indications for listing
Symptomatic heart failure with peak VO_2 between 11 and 16 mL/kg/min
In patient not using beta-blocker peak $VO_2 \leq 14$ is an indication for listing (Level of Evidence B)
In patient using beta-blocker peal $VO_2 \leq 12$ is an indication for listing (Level of Evidence B)
Recurrent or refractory heart failure symptoms unresponsive to maximal vasodilators and a flexible diuretic program
Recurrent unstable myocardial ischemic syndromes requiring multiple hospitalization and not amenable to coronary revascularization
Primary cardiac tumors without evidence of metastatic disease

Inadequate indications for listing
Left ventricular ejection fraction < 30% with mild to moderate symptoms
History of NYHA class IV symptoms or transient need for inotropic support on *suboptimal* medical regimen
Peak VO_2 > 16 mL/kg/min without other clinical indications
Prior life-threatening arrhythmias that are now controlled
Asymptomatic nonsustained ventricular tachycardia and advanced left ventricular dysfunction

Adopted from Ginns LC "Transplantation" Blackwell Science.

approximately less than 30%. The 1-year survival is between 30 and 80%, if VO_2max is between 10 and 18 and more than 80% for those patients with VO_2max greater than 18 mL/kg/min.[10] Currently patients should be considered as cardiac transplant candidate if VO_2max is below 14 mL/kg/min. In the patient taking a beta-blocker, a cutoff for peak VO_2 of $\leq$12 mL/kg/min should be used to guide listing. Both cutoffs are level of evidence B.[11] The group with VO_2max below 10 mL/kg/min would benefit most from cardiac transplantation. VO_2max between 10 and 14 in patients with major limitation of activities of daily living (ADL) are considered a probable indication for cardiac transplantation.

Contraindication

Presence of any condition that would shorten life expectancy or increase the risk of death from rejection or complications of immunosuppression is considered as a contraindication for cardiac transplantation. Detailed contraindications for cardiac transplant are listed in Table 10.2.

TABLE 10.2. Contraindications for cardiac transplantation

Absolute Contraindication
Age over 70 years (depends on the center)
Fixed pulmonary hypertension
Pulmonary vascular resistance greater than 5 Woods Unit
Transpulmonary gradient greater than 15 mmHg
Systemic illness that will limit survival despite heart transplant
Neoplasm other than skin. Five-year remission period is required. Low-grade prostate cancer that has not been "cured" (by prostate-specific antigen measurement) or in remission less than 5 years is generally recognized as a contraindication
HIV/AIDS (CD4 count less than 200 cells/mm^3)
Systemic lupus erythematosus or sarcoid that has multisystem involvement and is still active
Any systemic process with a high probability of recurring in the transplanted heart

Relative contraindications
Age over 65 years
Peripheral vascular disease not amenable to surgical or percutaneous therapy
Severe symptomatic cerebrovascular disease which is no amenable to revascularization
Severe pulmonary disease
Irreversible renal dysfunction – estimated glomerular filtration rate less than 40 mL/min
Diabetes mellitus with end-organ damage (neuropathy, nephropathy, retinopathy) or poor glycemic control (glycosylated hemoglobin [HbA1C > 7.5]) despite optimal control
Psychosocial impairment that jeopardizes the transplanted heart (antisocial personality disorder, medication noncompliance, drug or alcohol addictions, cigarette smoking, inability to rely on alternative care givers in the event of patient impairment)

Adopted from Steinman TI, Becker BN, Frost AE, Olthoff KM, Smart FW, Suki WN, Wilkinson AH Guidelines for the referral and management of patients eligible for solid organ transplantation. Clinical Practice Committee, American Society of Transplantation. Transplantation 71(9):1189–204, 2001.

(continued)

TABLE 10.2. (continued)

Edited with Mehra MR, Kobashigawa J, Starling R, Russell S, Uber PA, Parameshwar J, Mohacsi P, Augustine S, Aaronson K, Barr M. Listing criteria for heart transplantation. International Society for Heart and Lung Transplantation Guidelines for the Care of Cardiac Transplant Candidates. The Journal of Heart and Lung Transplantation.

United Network for Organ Sharing and Organ Allocation Criteria

In the United States, the system used for allocating organs for transplantation has been developed by the United Network for Organ Sharing (UNOS), a nonprofit organization that administers the Organ Procurement and Transplantation Network (OPTN). The OPTN was established in 1984, by the US Congress under the National Organ Transplant Act (NOTA) to unify transplant networks. Through the OPTN, the UNOS collect and manage data about every transplant event occurring in the United States, facilitate the organ matching and placement process, and develop transplantation policy. The UNOS status codes for cardiac transplantation medical urgency are shown in Table 10.3.[12]

TABLE 10.3. The UNOS status codes for medical urgency

Status 1A
Patient is admitted to the listing transplant center and has at least one of the following devices or therapies in place:
Mechanical support for acute hemodynamic decompensation that include at least one of the following:
Left or right ventricular device assist device implanted for 30 days or less (30 day period used at transplant center discretion)
Total artificial heart
Intra-aortic balloon pump
Extracorporeal membrane oxygenator
Mechanical circulatory support for more than 30 days with objective medical evidence of significant device-related complications such as thromboembolism, device infection, mechanical failure, and/ or life-threatening arrhythmias (may not require hospitalitation at transplant center)
Mechanical ventilation
Continuous infusion of a single high-dose intravenous inotrope or multiple intravenous inotropes, in addition to continuous hemodynamic monitoring of left ventricular filling pressures
Life-expectancy without heart less than 7 days

(continued)

TABLE 10.3. (continued)

Status 1B
A patient listed as Status 1B has at least one of the following devices or
  therapies in place:
  Left and/or right ventricular assist device implanted for more than 30
    days; or
  Continuous infusion of intravenous inotropes

Status 2
A patient who does not meet the criteria for Status 1A or 1B

Status 7
A patient listed as Status 7 is considered temporarily unsuitable to
  receive a thoracic organ transplant

Adapted from UNOS Web site http://www.unos.org/PoliciesandBylaws2/
policies/pdfs/policy_9.pdf.

EVALUATION OF PATIENT PRIOR CARDIAC TRANSPLANTATION

Baseline Tests in Transplant Candidate

Evaluation of the candidate for cardiac transplantation includes
complete history and physical examination. Laboratory test
should include blood chemistry including renal (BUN, creatinine, calcium, magnesium, phosphorus) and liver profiles
(bilirubin, alkaline phosphotase, AST, ALT), hematology, coagu-
lation tests, lipid profile, and urinalysis. Men should have prostate-
specific antigen (PSA) tested. In the case of diabetics or presence
of protein in urine, 24-h urine collection for creatinine clearance and/or protein collection and protein immunopheresis are
necessary. Patients should be screened for infectious diseases;
hepatitis A, B, and C virus; herpes virus; HIV; and cytomegalo-
virus (CMV). In addition to blood test, every candidate should
undergo pulmonary function test with arterial blood gases, and
stool for occult blood.[9]

Specific Blood Tests

Immunology studies include ABO blood type and antibody screen.
Panel reactive antibody (PRA) as well as HLA typing should be
performed. HLA typing assesses the presence of specific HLA antigens in the recipient. PRA is the examination of serum from a prospective transplant recipient for presence of circulating anti-HLA

antibodies. PRA establishes degree of humoral sensitization and it is represented as percentage of lymphocytes (representing the most common HLA antigens) against which the patient's serum reacts. A PRA greater than 10% is considered positive. It is suggested that positive PRA increases the incidence of posttransplant humoral type of rejection.[9]

Consultations

Every transplant candidate should undergo psychiatric, social, and nutritional evaluation. Dental and ophthalmoscopic examination should be performed.[9]

Imaging

Every patient should have abdominal ultrasound, carotid ultrasound, and chest X-ray (PA and lateral). Women should have mammography performed. The patients older than 50 or who are in the particular risk of atherosclerotic disease should undergo ankle brachial index evaluation.[9]

REJECTION

There are three types of graft rejection observed among heart transplant recipients: hyperacute rejection, acute cellular rejection, and vascular rejection.

Hyperacute Rejection

Hyperacute rejection is a *violent* immune response to the graft occurring immediately (minutes to hours after graft transplantation), caused by preexisting antibody against HLA epitopes or the ABO system. It almost always results in the loss of the organ. Hyperacute rejection could be prevented by the ABO compatibility and HLA matching.

Acute Cellular Rejection

Acute rejection is a cellular phenomenon, occurring days to months posttransplantation. The mononuclear inflammatory response against the graft is responsible for acute cellular rejection. The key histopathologic feature of this type of rejection is a presence of myocyte damage. The ISHLT grades rejection are as follows: Grade 0 R – no rejection, Grade 1 R, mild - interstitial and perivascular infiltrate up to one focus of myocyte damage, Grade 2 R, moderate – two or more foci of infiltrate with associated myocyte damage and Grade 3 R - diffuse infiltrate with myocyte damage and/or edema and/or hemorrhage and/or vasculititis.[13]

Chronic Rejection/Cardiac Allograft Vasculopathy

Cardiac allograft vasculopathy (CAV) is a unique form of obliterative coronary artery disease with unclear pathogenesis. Histopathologically CAV is characterized by concentric myointimal proliferation, diffusely involving the entire length of the coronary tree.[14–18]

IMMUNOSUPPRESSION THERAPY

Immune therapy is necessary to suppress the natural response of recipient to allograft, and it should be balanced between providing enough immunologic tolerance to allow acceptance of the transplanted heart and its adverse side effects. There are usually three situations which require specific combinations of immunosuppressive agents (1) high-dose initial immunosuppression to allow graft acceptance; (2) maintenance therapy for chronic acceptance of the graft; and (3) augmented immunosuppression to reverse acute rejection.

Induction Therapy

Induction therapy is an initial form of immunosuppressive therapy administered prior and/or early after transplantation. Its role is to induce the state of partial immune tolerance, increase initial global immunosuppression until maintenance of immunosuppression is achieved and facilitate the action of maintenance immunotherapy.

Maintenance (Baseline) Immunosuppression

Maintenance therapy is a form of immunosuppressive therapy administered chronically to ensure immune tolerance and chronic acceptance of the graft. The use of combinations of immunosuppressive drugs allows lower the dose of each medication (synergism) and decrease the risk of toxicity. There are there basic components of baseline immunosuppression (1) primary agent should be a calcineurin antagonist (blocks IL-2 production – the currently used agents are CsA or tacrolimus); (2) second agent should inhibit cellular replication and proliferation – currently used agents are azathioprine or more commonly now mycophenolate mofetil; and (3) use of corticosteroids, early posttransplant and taper down within first 6 months.

Augmented Immunosuppression to Reverse Acute Rejection

Augmented immunosuppression is a therapy aimed to reverse acute rejection of the graft. Depending on the stage of the rejection, it includes pulse dose of corticosteroids, adjusting the dose of baseline immunosuppressive therapy, cytolytic therapy with IV monoclonal antibodies, plasmapheresis, or adding cytotoxic therapy (methotraxate).

Immunosuppression Agents
Specific information regarding immunosuppressant is shown in Table 10.4.

INFECTIOUS COMPLICATION AFTER CARDIAC TRANSPLANTATION

Infectious complications observed in cardiac graft recipients could be divided accordingly to the time after the transplant and degree of immunosuppression. In general, during the first month of posttransplant the most common infections are the nosocomial bacterial or fungal infections of surgical wound, lungs, or indwelling vascular catheters: From first month till six months, the infectious complications are caused by immunomodulating viruses: CMV, EBV, HBV, or HCV. In addition, this is a time for appearance of the opportunistic infections with *Pneumocystis carinii*, aspergillus, and *Listeria monocytogenes*. After 6 months the infectious complications are similar to those among general population – pneumonia or viral infections. In the patients with recurrent rejection episodes and increased exposure to the immunosuppressive medications, the opportunistic infections with *P. carinii*, Cryptococcus, or Listeria might occur.[19]

MALIGNANCY

Malignancies in posttransplant patients can come from three major sources:

1. Preexisting malignancies that became clinically overt after the transplantation
2. Transmission of a malignancy from donor to recipient
3. De novo malignancy arising in the recipient following cardiac transplantation

Recurrence of preexisting malignancies. There are limited data in cardiac transplant, however, one study estimates that among heart and lung transplant patients with preexisting malignancies rate of recurrence or persistence of the malignancy was 19%. The neoplasms most likely to recur in heart, lung, and heart/lung recipients are lung cancer, nonmelanoma skin cancer, lymphomas, pancreatic and bladder cancer.

TABLE 10.4. Immunosupression Agents

Medication	Mechanisms of Action	Side Effects/Toxicities	Comments
Calcineurin inhibitors:			
Cyclosporine A (CsA)	Inhibits the calcineurin-dependent transcription through binding to the family of immunophilin-cyclophilin.	Nephrotoxicity hypertension hepatotoxicity metabolic acidosis hyperkalemia hyperlipidemia hyperuricemia excessive hair growth gingival hyperplasia.	Diltiazem increases the CsA level; metabolized by cytochrom P450, interactions with P450 inhibitors and inducers
Tacrolimus (Prograf)	Inhibits the calcineurin-dependent transcription through binding to the family of immunophilin – FK binding protein (FKBP) -12.	Nephrotoxicity, neurological effects: tremor, headache, insomnia, nightmares, rarely encephalopathy), glucose intolerance hyperkalemia Higher risk of Posttransplant Lymphoproliferative Disorder (PTLD).	about 100 times more potent than CsA
Corticosteroids:			
Prednisone Prednisolone	Immunosuppressive effects of steroid are due to impairment of transcription of specific genes encoding inflammatory cytokines	Glucose intolerance/diabetes mellitus Cushing syndrome impaired wound healing Osteoporosis cataracts hypertension	Majority of centers try to taper the dose of corticosteroids to every-other day low dose or no steroids by 3-6 months post-transplant.

Mycophenolate mofetil (Cellcept)	Prodrug, hydrolyzed to mycophenolic acid (MPA), which blocks the de novo pathway for purine synthesis and inhibition of DNA synthesis in human lymphocytes.	Gastrointestinal tract symptoms (nausea, vomiting, and diarrhea), dysuric symptoms and cholestasis.	Used in the maintenance therapy, often as substitution for azathioprine
Azathioprine (Imuran)	Nitroimidazole derivative of 6-mercaptopurine (6-MP); and as a purine analog impairs DNA synthesis and acts as an antiproliferative agent.	Dose-dependant myelosupression: leucopenia, thrombocytopenia and anemia (reversed by Dose reduction/ discontinuation) hepatotoxicity, pancreatitis, alopecia, megaloblastic anemia	Used as a maintenance therapy with corticosteroids and CsA/tacrolimus
Inhibitors of the target of rapamycin (TOR) enzyme – sirolimus/ everolimus	The mammalian target of rapamycin (mTOR) is phosphatidylinositol kinase like protein that plays important role in the process of T-cell activation. TOR-dependent activation is required for the cell to be effectively stimulated by the IL-2 to progress from the G1 phase into the S phase of the cell cycle, resulting in cell proliferation. Inhibitors of the target of rapamycin (TOR) enzyme – inhibit cytokine-mediated TOR-dependent cell division and proliferation. They have a synergistic effect with CsA.	Mild thrombocytopenia, mild anemia and dyslipidemia.	

(continued)

Table 10.4. (continued)

Medication	Mechanisms of Action	Side Effects/Toxicities	Comments
Monoclonal antibodies			
OTK-3	OTK3 is a murine monoclonal antibody with epitope specific for the CD3 complex. CD3 antigen is present on all mature T-lymphocytes and it is closely related to the antigen recognition site of the T-cell receptor. OTK3 administration results in depletion of CD3 cell from peripheral blood within 30-60 minutes, creating the state of immune tolerance.	Adverse effects include: cytokine release syndrome: fever, chills, headache, myalgias, increased susceptibility to CMV infections and Posttransplant Lymphoproliferative Disorder.	OTK3 are used in the induction therapy, steroid-resistant or recurrent rejection, and in rejection with hemodynamic compromise.
Anti-CD25 (Basiliximab, Daclizumab)	Monoclonal antibodies bind to the α–chain of the highly affinity IL-2 receptor on activated T-lymphocyte. They inhibit IL-2 –related proliferation of already activated T-lymphocytes.	Similar to OTK3	The use of anti-CD25 antibodies might be associated with fewer rejection episodes and longer interval to the first rejection episode.

Transplantation of a donor malignancy. There are case reports of transplantation of a donor malignancy, however; in the UNOS report of outcomes of the solid organ recipient, no donor transmitted recipient malignancy was identified.

De novo recipient malignancy. De novo malignancies are long-term complications of cardiac transplantation and chronic immunosuppression. Impaired immune surveillance in the course of immunosuppressive therapy, chronic foreign antigenic stimulation, synergistic effect of immunosuppressive agents and oncogens, impaired immunoregulation (in the case of lymphoid tumors), and oncogenic viruses play important role in the development of posttransplant malignancies.

Posttransplant Lymphoproliferative Disorder

Posttransplant lymphoproliferative disorder (PTLD) is defined as a presence of an abnormal proliferation of lymphoid cells, induced by EBV.[20–22] This includes both hyperplastic and neoplastic forms. Risk factors for PTLD include prolonged cytolytic therapy, CMV disease, and no pretransplant immunity to the EBV.[23] PTLD can present as an infectious mononucleosis-like illness, organ system involvement (allograft, GI tract, CNS, lungs, etc.), and as a disseminated disease. Primary therapy for PTLD is a reduction of immunosuppression. For localized disease, surgical resection is possible. For disease involving more than one anatomic site, chemotherapy is an option. If there is an evidence of circulating EBV, therapy with ganciclovir could be used. Additional modes of therapy include anti-B cell antibodies, interferon, and radiation. Prognosis depends on type of PTLD. Survival after diagnosis of lymphoma or lymphoproliferative disease ranges from 45 to 80% at 2 years. Multiorgan, late PTLD and CNS involvement are associated with worse outcome.

Different Types of Carcinomas

The most common type of tumors (40%) occurring among the transplant recipients are premalignant lesions (precancerous keratoses, Bowen's disease, and keratoacanthoma) and cutaneous carcinomas with squamous cell carcinoma being more frequent than basal cell carcinoma.[24] The most common noncutaneous malignancy is lung cancer usually occurring in patient with significant prior history of smoking. Other types of cancer seen among posttransplant patients are gastrointestinal cancers (oral cavity cancer, the esophagus, stomach, colon, and the rectal cancer), genitourinary tract carcinomas (kidney, urinary bladder, and in female cancers of the cervix, the vulva and vagina), and

TABLE 10.5. Routine surveillance for posttransplant patients

Test	Frequency
Stool for occult blood	Yearly (patients >50 years of age)
Colonoscopy alternating with flexible sigmoidoscopy	Every 3 years (patients >50 years of age)
Digital rectal exam	Yearly (males >50 years of age)
Prostate specific antigen	Every 2 years (males >50 years of age)
Mammogram	Yearly (females >35 years of age)
Pelvic exam and Pap smear	Yearly (females >35 years of age)
Chest X-ray	With each routine clinical visit (every 6 months)
Dermatology	Yearly
Lipid profile	Every 6–12 months
Bone density screening	Yearly
Ophthalmology exam	Yearly
Dental exam	Every 6 months

Adapted from Cleveland Clinic and UAB for detection of malignancy, hyperlipidemia, osteoporosis, and ocular complications.

thyroid gland. Overall the risk of cancer among the posttransplant patient is about fourfold increased as compared to the general population.[25]

Screening for Different Types of Cancers
Screening for malignancies is very important among posttransplant patients. Table 10.5 describes routine screening strategies among postheart transplant patients.

OTHER LONG-TERM POSTTRANSPLANT COMPLICATIONS
Hypertension
Arterial hypertension is a common clinical problem encountered among transplant recipients. The most common cause of posttransplant hypertension is a use of CsA (or tacrolimus). It is estimated that 40–90% of patients in CsA era are hypertensive as compared to only 20% in precyclosporine era.[26,27] CsA induces hypertension through different pathways: sympathetic stimulation, neurohormonal activation, and direct vascular effect. Other factors affecting the prevalence of hypertension are use of corticosteroids with direct effect on sodium retention and cardiac denervation. Therapy of HTN among posttransplant patient is very important and reflects similar goal as in general population. Sodium restriction is not efficient in posttransplant patients.

Calcium Channel Blockers

In pharmacological therapy, calcium channel blockers are the first line therapy, especially use of diltiazem results in lower dose of CsA. The dihydropyridine calcium channel blockers (such as amlodipine and felodipine) are frequently used as early antihypertensive agents due to minimal drug interactions in the posttransplant period.

Angiotensin Converting Enzyme Inhibitors

Other first line agents are angiotensin converting enzyme (ACE) inhibitors.

Diuretics

Diuretic therapy is also effective especially in the state of increased volume after the transplantation.

Alpha-Adrenergic Blocking Agents

Alpha-adrenergic blocking agents are useful in some patients.

Beta-Blocking Agents

Beta-blockers were traditionally avoided in cardiac transplant patients because of negative chronotropic effect and concern regarding inadequate heart rate response to exercise. This is especially true in the earlier posttransplant period. However, some patients might use carvedilol with its vasodilating effect. Other beta blockers are often used later after cardiac transplantation.

Hyperlipidemia

Corticosteroids and CsA are the most important agents contributing to development of hyperlipidemia.[28] CsA decreases bile acid synthesis from cholesterol, increasing cholesterol level, and directly (binds to LDL receptor) elevates the LDL level. In addition, CsA decreases activity of lipoprotein lipase, impairing clearance of VLDL and LDL. CsA levels inversely correlate with HDL level. Tacrolimus has similar effects on lipid as CsA, however, less pronounced. Prednisone increases free fatty acid synthesis, stimulates activity of 3-hydroxy 3-methylglutaryl coenzyme A (HMG-CoA) reductase, and inhibits lipoprotein lipase. These actions result in increased levels of VLDL, total cholesterol, and triglycerides, and in decreased levels of HDL.

HMG-CoA Reductase Inhibitors

Baseline therapy for hyperlipidemia in posttransplant patients is HMG-CoA reductase inhibitors ("statins"). Pravastatin has been proven to reduce cholesterol levels in cardiac transplant patients;

in addition reduced the incidence of rejection with hemodynamic compromise, decreased graft vasculopathy, and improved 1-year survival.[29]

Based on these data, pravastatin is routinely prescribed to all patients, early posttransplant irrespectively of lipid level, unless liver profile remains normal. Another agent studied in posttransplant patients was simvastatin. Rhabdomyolysis was observed among patients using statins and CsA, especially when they were taking niacin or gemfibrozil.

Bile Acid Sequestrants

Bile acid sequestrants can be used in posttransplant patients, but level of CsA should be closely monitored, because of interaction with CsA absorption.

Fibric Acid Derivatives

Gemfibrozil is most commonly used and indicated for marked hypertrigliceridemia. It should be avoided in combination with statins because of the risk of rhabdomyolysis.

Bone Complications

Osteoporosis

At 2-year posttransplantation, 28% patients had evidence of osteoporosis in the lumbar spine and 20% in the femoral neck. It is estimated that most of the bone density loss occurs with 6 months after cardiac transplant and is most prominent in the lumbar spine. Glucocorticosteroids, CsA, and renal insufficiency *are* thought to be responsible for development of osteoporosis.

Management of osteoporosis in posttransplant patients includes the following: routine annual screening for osteoporosis with bone mineral density measurements and elimination or minimization of corticosteroids, calcium and vitamin D3 supplementation, and biphosphonates.

Avascular Necrosis

Avascular necrosis of the bone is a condition characterized by disruption of blood supply to the bone with ischemia and subsequent necrosis of bone and cartilage. The prevalence of avascular necrosis among posttransplant patients is estimated between 3 and 6% (the most common bone the femoral head). The corticosteroids are responsible for this condition. Symptoms include pain, frequently at night and without weight bearing. Imaging studies confirmed the diagnosis with MRI being the most sensitive test.

Gastrointestinal Complications

Upper Gastrointestinal Disease
Disease of the esophagus. Esophagitis among transplant recipients result form *Candida albicans*, invasive CMV or HSV infection. The test of choice is an upper endoscopy.

Peptic ulcer disease (PUD). The invasive CMV, herpes (HSV) infection and chronic use of corticosteroids are the most important causes of the PUD among the posttransplant patients.

Cholelithiasis
Cyclosporine has been associated with the development of cholelithiasis among posttransplant patients.[30] Ursodeoxycholic acid is used to dissolve noncalcified gallstones but its efficacy is limited. Treatment of choice of symptomatic cholelithiasis is cholecystecomy; however, there are no data on asymptomatic cholelithiasis. Acalculous cholelithiasis has been reported among cardiac transplant and been associated with bile stasis and ischemia.

Pancreatitis
Pancreatitis in cardiac recipients has been associated with the following conditions: cholelithiasis, hyperlipidemia, invasive CMV disease, and medications such as azathioprine. Incidence of pancreatitis is low ranging 5–10%. The management of acute pancreatitis should be aggressive and similar to general population.

Diverticular Disease
Incidence of diverticular disease among transplant recipients is similar to those in general population but the complications (diverticulitis, abscess formation, and perforation) are unusual. Therapy of diverticulitis requires intravenous antibiotics, and perforation prompt surgery. Posttransplant patients might be more prone for perforation due to corticosteroid use.

References

1. Carrel A. The surgery of blood vessels. Johns Hopkins Hosp Bull 18:18, 1907
2. Sterioff S, Rucker-Johnson N, Frank C. Mann and transplantation at the Mayo Clinic. Mayo Clin Proc 62(11):1051–5, 1987
3. Mann FC, Priestley JT, Markowitz J, et al. Transplantation of the intact mammalian heart. Arch Surg 26:219, 1933
4. Goldberg A, Berman EVE, Akman OC. Homologous transplantation of the canine heart. J Int Coll Surg 30:575, 1958
5. Hardy JD, Kurrus FD, Chavez CM, Neely WA, Eraslan S, Turner MD, Fabian LW, Labecki TD. Heart transplantation in man. Developmental studies and report of a case. J Am Med Assoc 118:1132, 1964

6. Barnard CN. The operation. A human cardiac transplant: an interim report of a successful operation performed at Groote Schuur Hospital, Cape Town. S Afr Med J 41(48):1271–4, 1967

7. Taylor DO, Edwards LB, Boucek MM, Trulock EP, Deng MC, Keck BM, Hertz MI. Registry of the International Society for Heart and Lung Transplantation: twenty-second official adult heart transplant report - 2005. J Heart Lung Transplant 24(8):945–55, 2005

8. Taylor DO, Edwards LB, Boucek MM, Trulock EP, Aurora P, Christie J, Dobbels F, Rahmel AO, Keck BM, Hertz MI. Registry of the International Society for Heart and Lung Transplantation: twenty-fourth official adult heart transplant report – 2007. J Heart Lung Transplant 26(8):769–81, 2007

9. Mehra MR, et al. Listing criteria for heart transplantation: International Society for Heart and Lung Transplantation Guidline for the Care of Cardiac Transplant Candidates – 2006. J Heart Lung Transplant 25(9):1024–42, 2006

10. Mancin DM, Eisen H, Kussmaul W, Mull R, Edmunds LH Jr, Wilson JR. Value of peak exercise oxygen consumption for optimal timing of cardiac transplantation in ambulatory patients with heart failure. Circulation 83:778–86, 1991

11. http://www.jhltonline.org/article/PIIS1053249806004608/fulltext

12. http://www.unos.org/PoliciesandBylaws2/policies/pdfs/policy_9.pdf

13. Stewart S, Winters GL, Fishbein MC, Tazelaar HD, Kobashigawa J, Abrams J, Andersen CB, Angelini A, Berry GJ, Burke MM, Demetris AJ, Hammond E, Itescu S, Marboe CC, McManus B, Reed EF, Reinsmoen NL, Rodriguez ER, Rose AG, Rose M, Suciu-Focia N, Zeevi A, Billingham ME. Revision of the 1990 working formulation for the standardization of nomenclature in the diagnosis of heart rejection. J Heart Lung Transplant 24(11):1710–20, 2005

14. Uretsky BF, Murali S, Reddy PS, et al. Development of coronary artery disease in cardiac transplant patients receiving immunosuppressive therapy with cyclosporine and prednisone. Circulation 76:827, 1987

15. Pollack MS, Ballantyne CM, Patton-Ross C, et al. HLA match and other immunologic parameters in relation to survival, rejection severity and accelerated coronary artery disease after heart transplant. Clin Transplant 4:269, 1990

16. Tuzcu EM, De Franco AC, Goormastic M, et al. Dichotomous pattern of coronary atherosclerosis 1 to 9 years after transplantation: insights from systematic intravascular ultrasound imaging. J Am Coll Cardiol 27:839, 1996

17. Billingham ME. Graft coronary disease: the lesions and the patients. Transplant Proc 21:3665, 1989

18. Hiemann NE, Wellnhofer E, Knosalla C, et al. Prognostic impact of microvasculopathy on survival after heart transplantation: evidence from 9713 endomyocardial biopsies. Circulation 116:1274, 2007

19. Fishman JA. Infection in solid-organ transplant recipients. N Engl J Med 357(25):2601–14, 2007

20. Basgoz JP, Preiksaitis JK. P osttrasplant lymphoproliferative disorder. Infect Dis Clin North Am 9:901–23, 1995

21. Ho M, Miller G, Atchison RW, Breinig MK, Dummer JS, Andiman W, Starzl TE, Eastman R, Griffith BP, Hardesty RL, et al. Epstein-Barr virus infections and DNA hybridization studies in posttransplantation lymphoma and lymphoproliferative lesions; the role of primary infection. J Infect Dis 152(5):876-86, 1985

22. Nalesnik MA, Jaffe R, Starzl TE, Demetris AJ, Porter K, Burnham JA, Makowka L, Ho M, Locker J. The pathology of posttransplant lymphoproliferative disorders occurring in the setting of cyclosporine A-prednisone immunosuppression. Am J Pathol 133(1):173–92, 1988

23. Walker RC, Marshall WF, Strickler JG, Wiesner RH, Velosa JA, Habermann TM, McGregor CG, Paya CV. Pretransplantation assessment of the risk of lymphoproliferative disorder. Clin Infect Dis 20(5):1346-53, 1995

24. Couetil JP, McGoldrick JP, Wallwork J, English TA. Malignant tumors after heart transplantation. J Heart Transplant 9(6):622–6, 1990

25. Adami J, Gabel H, Lindelof B, Ekstrom K, Rydh B, Glimelius B, Ekbom A, Adami HO, Granath F. Cancer risk following organ transplantation: a nationwide cohort study in Sweden. Br J Cancer 89(7):1221–7, 2003.

26. Bennett WM, Porter JA. Cyclosporin-associated hypertension. Am J Med 85: 131–3, 1988

27. Chapman JR, Marcen R, Arias M, Raine AEG, Dunnill MS, Morris PJ. Hypertension after renal transplantation. Transplantation ;43:860–4, 1987

28. Kobashigawa JA, Kasiske BL. Hyperlipidemia in solid organ transplantation Transplantation 63(3):331–8, 1997

29. Kobashigawa JA, Katznelson S, Laks H, Johnson JA, Yeatman L, Wang XM, Chia D, Terasaki PI, Sabad A, Cogert GA, et al. Effect of pravastatin on outcomes after cardiac transplantation. N Engl J Med 333(10):621–7, 1995

30. Kahan BD, van Buren CT, Flechner SM, Jarowenko M, Yasumura T, Rogers AJ, Yoshimura N, LeGrue S, Drath D, Kerman RII. Clinical and experimental studies with cyclosporine in renal transplantation. Surgery 97(2):125–40, 1985

Chapter 11
Palliative Care and CHF

Aaron Olden and Timothy Quill

INTRODUCTION

The advanced heart failure disease trajectory is characterized by frequent exacerbations and disease remissions, which makes it difficult to prognosticate and to counsel patients considering more aggressive and invasive therapies. We explain how early palliative care intervention can help patients with advanced heart failure to understand disease course and maximize symptom control while continuing to pursue potentially beneficial disease-directed treatment. The management of pain and dyspnea in heart failure patients is discussed, and the similarities and differences between palliative care and hospice are explored. The reader will gain an understanding of the benefits of collaboration between palliative care providers and heart failure specialists such that health-related quality of life (HRQL) is maximized.

Background

The number of Americans living with heart failure is currently estimated to exceed five million, and despite significant advances in medical treatments, morbidity and mortality from this disease remain high.[13] The disease affects patients of all age groups, and is characterized by a slow, progressive course with frequent exacerbations and by impairments in quality of life and functional status. With modern treatment, patients with heart failure are now less likely to die suddenly and more likely to live longer with decreased functional capacity and more symptoms of chronic disease.

J.D. Bisognano et al. (eds.), *Manual of Heart Failure Management*,
DOI: 10.1007/978-1-84882-185-9_11, © Springer-Verlag London Limited 2009

For example, the recent introduction and widespread use of the implantable defibrillator has led to a reduction of sudden death mortality in those with heart failure, although reports have demonstrated that the HRQL is reduced in many of these patients.[9]

Health-Related Quality of Life and the Need for Palliative Care
Those living with heart failure suffer from reduced functional status and symptoms of pain, dyspnea, and depression (among others), and have been shown to receive more life-sustaining treatments than those with cancer.[11] Further, prognosis from heart failure is uncertain, and disease trajectory follows a more fluctuating course compared with other chronic diseases such as cancer or advanced dementia.[8]

Given this information, many have advocated involvement of palliative care services for those with heart failure from the time of first diagnosis,[5] not only to assist with pain and symptom management but also to help with communication, decision-making, and advance care planning. Patients with heart failure must often consider more invasive treatments such as implantable defibrillators and ventricular-assist devices, along with deciding whether or not to undergo resuscitation; some of these more aggressive treatments carry with them a significant impact on HRQL. Palliative care specialists can work together with patients and their cardiologists to help communicate disease course and prognosis, manage symptoms, as well as decide about more invasive treatments such that HRQL is maximized.

Outline
In this chapter, we will: (1) clearly define, compare, and contrast the services provided by palliative care specialists from those provided by hospice organizations; (2) illustrate how the disease trajectory and uncertain prognosis of those with heart failure make early palliative care intervention important; and (3) describe how palliative care specialists can help manage symptoms and maximize HRQL for those with heart failure as well as assist with medical decision-making.

PALLIATIVE CARE AND HOSPICE

Two Similar Yet Different Approaches
Many physicians and other health care providers may be unfamiliar with the services offered by specialists in palliative care and with the similarities/differences between hospice and palliative care.

Palliative specialists strive to provide relief from symptoms associated with chronic disease as well as assist both patients and families with the decision-making process surrounding such diseases. The approach is interdisciplinary – involving professionals from many fields including (but not limited to) physicians, nurses, social workers, and chaplains. The goal of the interdisciplinary group is to maximize quality of life while supporting patients and families in the context of their values and preferences. This philosophy of palliative care can occur at any point in the disease process; heart failure patients can continue to pursue active disease treatment including cardiac transplant with an understanding that relief of pain and other disease-related symptoms is as important as treatment of their underlying disease.

In contrast to palliative care, hospice services are a Medicare benefit in addition to a philosophy of care for those patients who have chosen to forego curative therapies and have shifted focus exclusively toward enhancing quality of life. Patients admitted to hospice programs receive both nursing and health aide services in the most suitable location (most commonly at home, but can also supplement care at a nursing home and elsewhere) as well as full coverage for medications and hospitalization, if needed to palliate symptoms. The hospice benefit requires that the patient's physician estimates that he or she is more likely than not to die in the next six months.

This distinction between hospice and palliative care is important, as many patients with heart failure who do not qualify for hospice services clearly stand to benefit from the palliative care approach. Many heart failure patients are not likely enough to die in the next six months to qualify for hospice, and many still stand to benefit from active disease-directed treatment. Palliative care philosophy allows for continued active disease-directed treatment, but simultaneously provides interdisciplinary expertise to maximize symptom relief and functional status. The ideal situation for heart failure patients would be early involvement of palliative care teams to maximize HRQL at the same time as they are receiving state-of-the-art disease-directed heart failure treatment, with a transition to hospice as disease-directed treatment options become ineffective.

DISEASE TRAJECTORY AND PROGNOSIS

Disease Trajectory
Some have found it helpful to use disease trajectories to assist with decision-making surrounding more invasive treatments and

consideration of hospice services. For example, those with cancer generally have a disease trajectory characterized by a steady but slow decline, followed by a more precipitous decrease in function and increase in symptoms as death approaches (Figure 11.1, top). This precipitous functional decline has traditionally been the point at which physicians and patients consider admission to hospice.

Disease trajectories for those with heart failure are not as predictable, creating a dilemma for heart failure clinicians. As illustrated in Figure 11.1 (middle), the heart failure trajectory is characterized by frequent disease exacerbations and remissions including visits to the emergency department and/or hospital admission for medication adjustment, diuresis, or more aggressive therapy, with a gradual functional decline over time. There is considerable prognostic uncertainty associated with this trajectory. In fact, on the day before a heart failure patient's death, it is often difficult to distinguish by clinical criteria from other heart failure patients who will live months or even years. Thus, in addition to a high prevalence of pain, dyspnea, anxiety, and depression, heart failure patients have considerable uncertainty about their future, which makes involvement of palliative care specialists early in the disease course potentially quite helpful. This also allows for periodic revisitation of preferences regarding end-of-life care in the context of continued active disease treatment, and may even minimize hospitalizations and exacerbations of the disease.

Prognosis
The unpredictable disease trajectory of those with heart failure makes it equally difficult to estimate and give accurate prognostic information to patients and families. Indicators such as hyponatremia, ventricular dilation, and maximal oxygen consumption are reliable markers for prognosis, but functional capacity remains one of the best predictors of mortality.[7] Most patients also struggle with this prognostic uncertainty and may simply understand that the disease follows a chronic course with the possibility of frequent exacerbations and the constant possibility of sudden death. The SUPPORT (Study to Understand Prognosis and Preferences for Outcomes and Results of Treatment) project illustrated that patients with cancer and heart failure use their own prognostic estimates to guide resuscitation decisions,[3] which emphasizes the need for communication of prognosis (however uncertain it may be) between physicians and patients on a regular basis.

We recommend that physicians caring for those with heart failure ask patients regularly how much information they desire regarding prognosis, and provide the best estimates possible such that patients can make educated decisions about further treatments

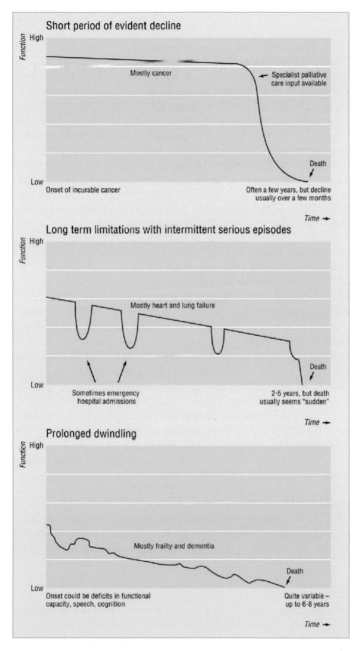

FIGURE 11.1. Trajectories of chronic disease. Used with permission: RAND Health, 2003.

and whether or not to place limits on more aggressive therapies. A prognostic estimate such that patients are given a range ("*A majority of patients with your current condition will live six months to a year...*") but with qualifiers on each end ("*...but every individual is different, so some will live less and others may live considerably longer*") can be very helpful to patients. Although this range is an estimate, it allows patients to prepare for the future and be sure that the remaining time they have is maximized. Physicians should also ask patients with heart failure about resuscitation preferences during outpatient visits whenever time permits and revisit such discussions when possible, especially if functional status starts to decline or if the patient is having frequent exacerbations. Palliative care specialists may be helpful in discussing therapeutic options with patients when prognosis is more uncertain and goals of treatment have not been well-defined.

MAXIMIZING QUALITY OF LIFE

Health-Related Quality of Life
How does heart failure affect quality of life and functional status? HRQL encompasses both of these terms. HRQL means "the functional effect of an illness and its consequent therapy on the patient, as perceived by the patient."[2] Thus, rather than "quality of life," which refers to the known effects of a *disease* on a patient, HRQL takes into account the *experience of the illness*,[6] including therapies, medication effects, and hospitalizations. Regularly revisiting symptom progression and functional status with both patients and their families and loved ones is the best approach to assessing HRQL. Using this concept of HRQL, the physician will be reminded that treatments and therapies, in addition to known effects of the disease itself, are likely to contribute both positively and negatively on the patient's overall illness experience.

Pain and Symptom Management[*]
Precise incidences of symptoms experienced by those with heart failure differ among reported studies, but it is well known that moderate to severe symptoms are common and their burden

---

*Here, we will briefly review the most common symptoms affecting heart failure patients, and refer the reader to the Primer of Palliative Care [10] for more information about these and other symptoms not discussed in this chapter.

increases as the disease progresses. Reported symptoms of those with heart failure include pain, dyspnea, depression, anxiety, anorexia, and nausea, among others. Although dyspnea is commonly considered a hallmark of heart failure exacerbations, (not to mention the symptom on which the New York Heart Association classification is based), pain affects up to 80% of patients with heart failure and is more common than dyspnea in some series.[12] Furthermore, psychological symptoms including anxiety and depression are common (present in up to one-third of heart failure patients) and are often the most distressing to patients. They deserve special consideration because they are so amenable to treatment. Physicians caring for patients with heart failure should regularly explore a "palliative review of systems" using a reliable scale like the Edmonton Symptom Assessment Scale,[1] and should also inquire about activities that are important to them, such as shopping and other social activities, to be sure that all aspects of HRQL are explored.

Treatment of Pain

Pain affects about 70–80% of heart failure patients. Pain may be ischemic, or related to other chronic illnesses such as osteoarthritis or neuropathy. Whatever the cause, pain symptoms should be further explored to determine whether the origin is somatic, visceral, or neuropathic, which will then help guide proper diagnosis and treatment. Nonsteroidal antiinflammatory agents (NSAIDS) should be generally avoided in patients with heart failure, as they can impair renal function, cause sodium retention, and possibly lead to hospitalization.

Patients should be asked to rate pain on a 0–10 scale, with 0 indicating no pain and 10 being the worst pain imaginable. For most patients, the goal should be to reduce pain to a level below 5 (a "mild" zone). Since NSAIDS are relatively contraindicated, acetaminophen may be the best choice when pain is mild. But when pain is moderate to severe, opioids remain the drugs of choice for pain relief for those with heart failure. When moderate to severe pain is chronic, short-acting opioids are first started on an every 4-hour basis with "as-needed" doses in between. When an effective total daily dose has been determined, the patient can be transitioned to a longer-acting preparation for more sustained pain relief throughout the day, with "as-needed" doses of short-acting preparations in between for breakthrough symptoms. For patients with renal failure, morphine should be avoided, as its metabolites can accumulate and lead to altered mental status and/or coma. Other opioids that are excreted by the liver should be substituted in equianalgesic doses. Palliative care specialists should be consulted in cases where pain has been difficult to control.

Treatment of Dyspnea

Dyspnea is also a common symptom in patients with heart failure, and is used in the NYHA classification of heart failure as an indicator of disease severity and progression. Thus, as the disease worsens, shortness of breath is present not only during activity but with minimal exertion or, as with Class IV failure, at rest. Patients with heart failure should be asked at each visit about shortness of breath, including its prevalence throughout the day and severity on a rating scale of 0–10 (similar to that for reporting pain). The experience of dyspnea may differ from one patient to another, so self-report on this 10 point scale over time can be a much more reliable measure of distress for a given patient than respiratory rate or oxygen saturation.

As with other symptoms, reversible causes of dyspnea should always be sought and treated, such as a therapeutic thoracentesis for pleural effusion and/or increased diuresis for pulmonary edema. In concert with such efforts, addition of palliative medications should be considered. Opioids are generally the first choice medication for the symptomatic treatment of dyspnea, as they are effective at suppressing the sensation of shortness of breath. Low doses of morphine, either in oral or parenteral form, can be considered first; if renal insufficiency is present, low-dose hydromorphone is more appropriate. Doses should be titrated upward with a goal of lessening dyspnea into the mild zone (<5 out of 10). If patients cannot rate dyspnea on a numeric scale, monitoring of facial expressions or respiratory rate should be considered. Strategies for initiating and then titrating opioids for dyspnea are similar to the approach to pain management as outlined earlier.

Sometimes the anxiety associated with being short of breath is relieved by treating the dyspnea with opioids. Any anxiety that remains after the dyspnea has been fully treated should be addressed with additional measures. Benzodiazepines are helpful in this latter circumstance; oral lorazepam is a good first choice as it has a short half-life and can be used as needed for anxiety or in scheduled doses if the symptom is more distressing and persistent. Relaxation techniques and creating an environment with clean, circulating air are also helpful with these symptoms.

Treatment of Other Symptoms

Readers are referred to the *Primer of Palliative Care* for more information about the management of these and other symptoms.[10] The prevalence of anxiety and depression, although not discussed in detail above, is high in this population, so screening for these symptoms should be performed at each visit. Collaboration with palliative care providers should be considered from the time of diagnosis to ensure that HRQL is maximized while continuing to pursue the best possible disease-directed treatment.

END-OF-LIFE DECISION-MAKING AND HOSPICE

Variable disease trajectories and uncertain prognosis for heart failure account in part for the difficulty with developing clear criteria for hospice admission in these patients. Nevertheless, the National Hospice and Palliative Care Organization has developed hospice admission criteria for heart failure patients (Box 11.1). In general, a continued functional decline and an ejection fraction less than 20% in spite of maximal disease-directed therapy is required.

Box 11.1. National Hospice and Palliative Care Organization General Medical Guidelines for Determining Prognosis in Selected Noncancer Diseases*

The Patient Should Meet All of the Following Criteria

  I. The patient's condition is life limiting, and the patient and/ or family knows this.

 II. The patient and/or family have elected treatment goals directed toward relief of symptoms rather than the underlying disease.

III. The patient has either of the following:

   A. Documented clinical progression of the disease, which may include

      1. Progression of the primary disease process as listed in the disease-specific criteria, as documented by serial physician assessment and laboratory, radiologic, or other studies.

      2. Multiple emergency department visits or inpatient hospitalizations over the prior 6 months.

      3. For homebound patients receiving home health services, nursing assessment may be documented.

      4. For patients who do not qualify under 1,2, or 3, a recent decline in functional status should be documented. Clinical judgement is required.

   B. Documented recent impaired nutritional status related to the terminal process:

      1. Unintentional, progressive weight loss of more than 10% over the prior 6 months.

(continued)

Box 11.1. (continued)

---

   2. Serum albumin <2.5 g/dL may be a helpful prognostic indicator but should not be used in isolation from other factors above.

Patients With Heart Disease Should Also Meet the Following Criteria

   I. Intractable or frequently recurrent symptomatic heart failure or intractable angina pectoris with heart failure.
   II. Patient's should already be optimally treated with diuretics, vasodilators, β–blockers, and spironolactone as indicated and tolerated.[†]
   III. Other factors contributing to a poor prognosis: symptomatic arrhythmias, history of cardiac arrest and resuscitation or syncope, cardiogenic brain embolism, or concomitant HIV disease.

---

*Adapted with permission from National Hospice Organization.[00]
[†]This criterion is modified from the published guideline to reflect current, optimal medical management of heart failure.

It is necessary to document this clinical progression – including a decline in performance status and frequent hospitalizations and/or emergency room visits. Each downward trend in performance status should be taken as an opportunity for patients, families, and their physicians to discuss their willingness to pursue or forego more aggressive and invasive treatments [such as implantable defibrillators, ventricular-assist devices, and/or cardiopulmonary resuscitation (CPR)]. Potential benefits and burdens of these more invasive therapies should be discussed with patients not only with respect to how they may prolong life but also how they might affect HRQL. Withholding more invasive treatments in patients with advanced symptoms should be considered if the likelihood for meaningful improvement in HRQL is minimal.

Forty percent of advanced heart failure patients over age 64 would prefer a do-not-resuscitate (DNR) status,[4] yet DNR orders are often not completed until the last days of life if at all. Patients should be educated about the likelihood of resuscitation being successful, and patients' wishes with regard to CPR should be explored while cognitive status is still intact. This allows the burden of decision-making to be shifted away from families and loved ones and can assure health care providers that patient' wishes are respected – a particularly important tenet in palliative and end-of-life care.

CONCLUSION

The care of patients with heart failure is both rewarding and challenging. Recent advances in the field of cardiology and cardiac surgery have improved mortality for heart failure patients, although decision-making around these treatments has become more complex. Challenges of ensuring informed consent in the face of uncertainty about prognosis and treatment utility can be countered by collaboration with palliative care specialists early in the disease course, such that symptom control is optimized and patients' preferences regarding more invasive treatments in the future are fully explored and documented. In most cases, common symptoms that afflict heart failure patients such as pain and dyspnea can be controlled as can depression and anxiety. Communication with patients and their families is paramount at all stages of heart failure, and should address both benefits and burdens of therapy as well as potential effects of such therapy on HRQL. This allows for a shared decision-making, and ensures that patients' wishes are respected while HRQL is optimized.

References

1. Bruera E, Kuehn N et al. et al. (1991). The Edmonton Symptom Assessment System (ESAS): a simple method for the assessment of palliative care patients. Journal of Palliative Care 7:6–9.
2. Coelho R, Ramos S et al. (2005). Heart failure and health related quality of life. Clin Pract Epidemol Ment Health 1:19.
3. Covinsky KE, Fuller JD et al. (2000). Communication and decision-making in seriously ill patients: findings of the SUPPORT project. The Study to Understand Prognoses and Preferences for Outcomes and Risks of Treatments. J Am Geriatr Soc 48:S187–93.
4. Formiga F, Chivite C et al. (2004). End-of-life preferences in elderly patients admitted for heart failure. QJM 97:803–8.
5. Gibbs JS, McCoy AS et al. (2002). Living with and dying from heart failure: the role of palliative care. Heart 88 Suppl 2:ii36–9.
6. Guyatt GH et al. (1993). Measurement of health-related quality of life in heart failure. JACC 22(4); 185A–191A.
7. Hauptman PJ, Havranek EP et al. (2005). Integrating Palliative Care into Heart Failure Care. Arch Intern Med 165: 374–8.
8. Murray SA, Kendall M et al. (2005). Illness trajectories and palliative care. BMJ 330:1007–11.
9. Noyes K, Corona E et al. (2007). Health-related quality of life consequences of implantable cardioverter defibrillators: results from MADIT II. Med Care 45:377–85.
10. Quill T et al. (2007). Primer of Palliative Care, 4th ed. American Academy of Hospice and Palliative Medicine, Illinois.

11. Tanvetyanon T, Leighton JC et al. (2003). Life-sustaining treatments in patients who died of chronic congestive heart failure compared with metastatic cancer. Crit Care Med 31:60–4.
12. Ward C et al. (2002). The need for palliative care in the management of heart failure. Heart 87:294–8.
13. Wilson JF et al. (2007). In the Clinic. Heart failure. Ann Intern Med 147:ITC12-1–ITC12-16.

Chapter 12
Device Therapy in Heart Failure

Mehmet Aktas and Spencer Rosero

IMPLANTABLE CARDIOVERTER DEFIBRILLATORS

Although medical therapy including ACE-inhibitors and beta-blockers have significantly reduced morbidity and mortality in patients with heart failure, these patients continue to suffer and are at particular risk for sudden cardiac death often due to ventricular tachyarrhythmias. The miniaturization of sophisticated machines such as cardiac pacemakers and defibrillators over the past 20 years has made device-based therapy an adjunctive therapeutic modality for patients with heart failure. A number of large, multicenter randomized clinical trials have demonstrated that device therapy in addition to optimal medical therapy can significantly reduce mortality and morbidity.

SUDDEN CARDIAC DEATH

Sudden death accounts for nearly 400,000 deaths in the overall United States population each year.[1] Nearly half the deaths in the heart failure population are sudden cardiac deaths. The risk of sudden death in the heart failure population is ninefold higher with an annual sudden death risk of 25% per year.[2] To date, use of anti-arrhythmics have failed to decrease the sudden death risk, and in fact several studies suggest increased risk with their use.[3,4] Patients with heart failure may experience nonsustained and sustained ventricular tachycardia, which can degenerate into ventricular fibrillation resulting in death. Implantable cardioverter defibrillators (ICD) implanted in patients without a history of sudden cardiac death or ventricular tachyarrhythmias are for primary

J.D. Bisognano et al. (eds.), *Manual of Heart Failure Management*,
DOI: 10.1007/978-1-84882-185-9_12, © Springer-Verlag London Limited 2009

prevention purposes. Patients who have survived a cardiac arrest or a life-threatening tachyarrhythmia receive an ICD for secondary prevention purposes.

ISCHEMIC CARDIOMYOPATHY

Patients with left ventricular dysfunction from ischemic heart disease due to myocardial infarction are at increased risk for sudden cardiac death from ventricular tachyarrhythmias. In the second Multicenter Automatic Defibrillator Implantation Trial (MADIT II), patients with a left ventricular ejection fraction <30% were randomized to either standard medical therapy or standard medical therapy and ICD implant at 30-day post myocardial infarction.[5] The trial was terminated early, because at a mean follow-up time of 20 months, patients randomized to the ICD arm had a significant lowering of all-cause mortality (14.2% vs. 19.8%, hazard ration 0.65, 95% confidence interval 0.51–0.93).

NONISCHEMIC CARDIOMYOPATHY

Patients with nonischemic cardiomyopathy are also at risk of sudden cardiac death. In the SCD-Heft trial, 2,521 patients with a left ventricular ejection fraction of <35% were randomized to ICD implantation, amiodarone therapy, or placebo.[6] Patients with nonischemic cardiomyopathy constituted 48% of the patients, while the remainder had ischemic cardiomyopathy. At five years, patients with ICDs had a significant lowering of overall mortality (29% vs. 36% with placebo, hazard ratio 0.77, 95% confidence interval 0.62–0.96), and the benefit of an ICD were comparable in those with either ischemic or nonischemic cardiomyopathy.

GUIDELINES FOR ICD IMPLANT

On the basis of these two pivotal trials and several others, the American College of Cardiology and the American Heart Association have published joint guidelines for ICD use in patients with heart failure.[7] ICD therapy is considered a Class I indication for the prevention of sudden cardiac death in patients with left ventricular dysfunction due to prior myocardial infarction (MI), who are 40 days post MI, who have an LVEF <30–40%, NYHA functional class II or III symptoms while on optimal medical therapy and have at least a one-year expected survival. Similarly, ICD therapy is a Class I indication for prevention of sudden cardiac death in patients with nonischemic cardiomyopathy, LVEF ≤30–35%, NYHA functional class II or III symptoms while on optimal medical and have at least a one-year expected survival.

ICD IMPLANTATION AND TESTING

Modern day ICD implants are performed by cardiac electrophysiologists in specialized laboratories. ICD implants are typically implanted in the left pectoral region and leads are placed transvenously with access either through the cephalic vein, axillary vein, or subclavian vein. In younger patients, and in patients who do not require pacing, a single chamber right ventricular lead is placed, and the ICD is typically programmed with a back-up ventricular pacing rate of 40 beats per minute (bpm) (Figure 12.1). Patients who have an indication for an ICD and for occasional pacing a dual chamber ICD is commonly implanted for both right atrial and right ventricular pacing to maintain atrioventricular synchrony. Most implanting electrophysiologists test the ICD at the time of implant, which is known as defibrillation threshold (DFT) testing. Once the device and leads are implanted, ventricular fibrillation is induced and the ICD is allowed to detect the tachyarrhythmia and

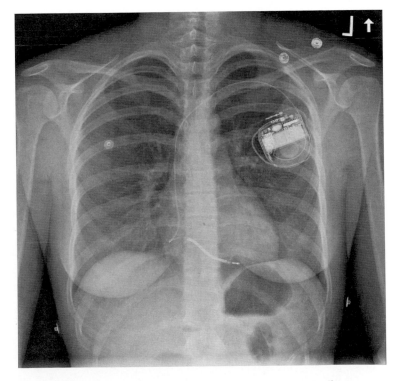

FIGURE 12.1. Single chamber implantable cardioverter defibrillator.

deliver therapy. Therefore, it is critical for these patients to be optimized from an electrolyte, ischemia and heart failure standpoint prior to undergoing DFT testing.

ICD PROGRAMMING

On the basis of the patients' functional class and clinical arrhythmia history, an ICD can be programmed to deliver a variety of different therapies to treat ventricular arrhythmias. ICD manufacturers have developed sophisticated algorithms that are used to identify a given arrhythmia. These algorithms attempt to identify arrhythmias based on tachycardia rate, duration, morphology, and regularity. Once a tachyarrhythmia is identified an ICD may deliver anti-tachycardia pacing (ATP) in attempt to overdrive pace the arrhythmia (Figure 12.2). If this fails the ICD may proceed to defibrillate the heart. Modern ICDs can be programmed to several zones of therapy, and within each zone a variety of different ICD therapies maybe included. For example, a typical ICD program may be programmed to a VT 1 zone for VT with a rate of 156–176 bpm, VT 2 zone for VT with a rate of 177–189 bpm and a VF zone for ventricular tachyarrhythmias with a rate >189 bpm. Often the initial therapy for VT falling in VT 1 and VT 2 zone will include ATP and if this fails to restore normal rhythm then the ICD therapy will proceed to include shocks with increasing energy levels. Current ICDs also log activity level and indirectly measure volume status, which may be used by treating clinicians to guide therapy or to gauge response to therapy.

ICD FOLLOW-UP AND MANAGEMENT

Once an ICD is implanted, patients are seen regularly in a device clinic to assure normal ICD generator and lead function, and to assess for symptomatic and asymptomatic as well as sustained and nonsustained arrhythmias. Device interrogation may reveal important clinical information, such as asymptomatic atrial fibrillation, which may require anticoagulation and titration of medical therapy. In addition to an in office ICD check, modern ICDs may also be interrogated while a patient is at home through specialized equipment using telephone lines. This home interrogation may be provided on a regular scheduled basis, or upon development of symptoms. The patient can then transmit an interrogation of the ICD and the clinician can review this interrogation through a secure, password protected internet Web site.

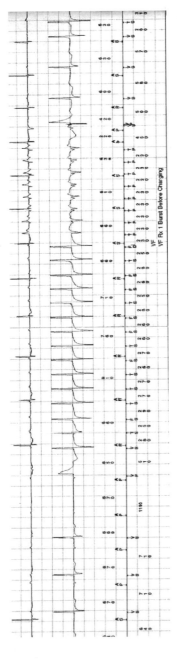

FIGURE 12.2. Rhythm strip from a device interrogation showing an episode of ventricular fibrillation (VF). Patient is initially atrial paced but suddenly develops VF. The arrhythmia is detected and while the device charges to deliver a shock, anti-tachycardia pacing is delivered, which terminates VF thereby averting the shock. The annotation on the bottom of the strip is the interpretation of the rhythm by the device. *TS* Tachy Sensed; *FS* Fibrillation Sensed; *TP* Tachy Pace; *AP* Atrial Pace; *VS* Ventricular Sense; *VP* Ventricular Paced.

ELECTRICAL STORM

Electrical storm, also known as arrhythmia storm or ventricular storm, is generally defined as the occurrence of 3 or more VT or VF episodes within a 24-h period. Each episode is usually separated by at least 5 min and requires consecutive high energy ICD shocks. Triggers for electrical storm are often worsening heart failure, electrolyte disturbances, and/or ischemia but are often unknown. Regardless of the mechanism, these patients have very significant short and long-term mortality.

ICD AND DRIVING

Patients who have an ICD are not allowed to drive commercial motor vehicles according the United States Department of Transportation's Federal Motor Carrier Safety Administration.[8] In February 2007, the American Heart Association and the Heart Rhythm Society published updated guidelines regarding personal driving in patients with ICDs.[9] According to these guidelines, patients receiving an ICD for primary prevention should be restricted from driving for at least the first week after ICD implant in order to allow healing and recovery. Patients receiving an ICD for secondary prevention and patients who receive appropriate ICD therapy, even if implanted initially for primary prevention, should avoid driving for a period of at least 6 months.

CARDIAC RESYNCHRONIZATION THERAPY (CRT)

Patients with heart failure often have electrocardiographic evidence of intraventricular conduction delay (IVCD), either right bundle branch block (RBBB) or left bundle branch block (LBBB). Patients with IVCD have dyssynchronous activation of the heart thereby compromising the hearts pumping ability. For example, patients with LBBB have delayed mechanical activation of the left ventricular free wall resulting in a nonuniform contraction of the heart with certain areas of the myocardium contracting while other areas remain relaxed. The loss of normal rapid synchronous electrical and mechanical activation of the myocardium may result in a lower left ventricular ejection fraction and lower cardiac output. Several studies have demonstrated that cardiac resynchronization therapy achieved through biventricular pacing improves contractility, left ventricular function, patients' functional class, and their overall risk of death.

Companion

In the Comparison of Medical Therapy, Pacing, and Defibrillation in Chronic Heart Failure (COMPANION) trial, 1,520 patients with

NYHA class III or IV heart failure, QRS $\geq$ 120 ms, LVEF $\leq$ 35%, and heart failure hospitalization within the past year were randomized to optimal medical therapy alone, CRT alone, or CRT with an ICD (CRT-D).[10] At a mean follow-up period of 12 months, a significant reduction in the composite primary end point of all-cause mortality and all-cause hospitalization occurred in both the CRT arms compared with the group receiving optimal medical therapy alone (56% and 56% vs. 68%, HR 0.80, 95% CI 0.68–0.95). The CRT-D arm showed a significant reduction in the secondary end point of all cause mortality whereas only a trend toward a mortality benefit was seen with the CRT only arm.

Care-hf
The Cardiac Resynchronization in Heart Failure (CARE-HF) trial randomized 813 patients with NYHA class III or IV heart failure, an LVEF $\leq$ 35%, and QRS $\geq$ 120 ms to cardiac resynchronization therapy with biventricular pacing or medical therapy alone.[11] At a mean of 29 months, CRT significantly reduced the time to death from any cause or unplanned hospitalization for a major cardiovascular event (39% vs. 55%, Hazard Ratio 0.63, 95% CI 0.51–0.77) and a significant mortality reduction was also observed with CRT (20% vs. 30%, HR 0.64%, 95% CI 0.48–0.85).

GUIDELINES FOR CRT
On the basis of these two pivotal trials and others, the American College of Cardiology and the American Heart Association recommend the use of CRT in the treatment of adult patients with chronic heart failure.[12] Use of cardiac resynchronization therapy is considered a Class I indication in patients with LVEF $\leq$ 35%, NYHA class III or IV heart failure despite optimal medical therapy, and who have dyssynchrony (defined as a QRS > 120 ms).

CRT IMPLANT AND PROGRAMMING
Biventricular pacing differs from conventional dual chamber pacing in that a third pacing lead is positioned in a branch of the coronary sinus so as to achieve left ventricular pacing (Figure 12.3). This multi-site pacing serves to reestablish atrioventricular, interventricular, and intraventricular synchrony. In rare cases where the left ventricular lead cannot be positioned through a transvenous approach, referral to a cardiac surgeon may be considered for epicardial left ventricular lead placement. Most cotemporary cardiac resynchronization devices also work as ICDs (CRT-D), since most of these patients also qualify for ICD implant for the above-mentioned reasons. Unlike standard pacemakers

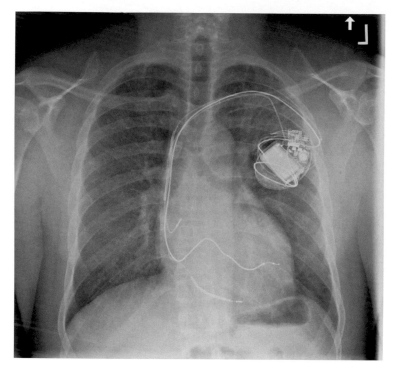

FIGURE 12.3. Biventricular Implantable Cardioverter Defibrillator. Three leads are seen, one each for right atrial pacing, right ventricular pacing and one in the coronary sinus for left ventricular pacing.

used for bradycardia indications where chronic right ventricular pacing may lead to heart failure, maximum benefit from CRT is realized with maximum biventricular pacing. Regular device monitoring and programming is performed to assure biventricular pacing is occurring. Depending on the underlying intraventricular delay (LBBB or RBBB), the timing for RV and LV pacing may be adjusted so as to achieve maximal hemodynamic improvement. Echocardiography may be used to help determine optimal timing settings for the atrioventricular delay, and for RV and LV pacing timing which is referred to as AV optimization.

FUTURE APPLICATIONS OF CRT
The University of Rochester Medical Center is conducting a large multicenter randomized clinical trial of CRT-D (MADIT-CRT) in patients with LVEF < 30%, QRS > 130 ms and NYHA class I or II

heart failure to determine if early cardiac resynchronization can halt the progression to advanced heart failure and reduce overall mortality.[13] MADIT-CRT has completed enrollment and patients are being followed for the primary endpoint. MADIT-CRT results will not be available for several years.

PERMANENT PACEMAKERS

Conduction abnormalities including atioventricular (AV) block, tachy-brady syndrome, and symptomatic bradycardia are common in patients with heart failure and may require a permanent pacemaker. Furthermore, effective therapy in patients with left ventricular dysfunction often requires medicines (e.g., beta-blockers, digoxin, amiodarone, sotalol) that may contribute to chronotropic incompetence and/or conduction abnormalities requiring a permanent pacemaker. Contemporary permanent pacemakers offer dual chamber (atrial and right ventricular) pacing and can be programmed to deliver pacing in a variety of different modalities (Table 12.1). Most pacemakers have built in accelerometers used to determine patient activity allowing physiologic regulation of heart rate response.

CHALLENGES OF CARDIAC PACING

Although cardiac pacing is available if necessary, chronic right ventricular pacing has deleterious hemodynamic effects particularly in patients with left ventricular dysfunction. Right ventricular pacing produces paradoxical septal motion and leads to intraventricular dyssynchrony such as in patients with left bundle branch block. The Dual Chamber and VVI Implantable Defibrillator (DAVID) trial randomized 506 ICD recipients with LVEF ≤ 40%, who had no indications for cardiac pacing to dual chamber pacing (DDDR 70) versus back-up ventricular pacing at 40 bpm (VVI 40).[15] The hypothesis was that dual chamber pacing would facilitate optimal medical therapy for heart failure, improve hemodynamics, and ultimately reduce heart failure hospitalization. At one year, the rate of death or hospitalization for heart failure was significantly higher for the group randomized to DDDR pacing compared with the group randomized to back up ventricular pacing only (26.7% vs. 16.1%, $p = 0.03$). This paradoxical increase in mortality and heart failure hospitalization was contributed primarily to "forced" right ventricular pacing in the group randomized to DDDR pacing. Our understanding of the negative hemodynamic effects of chronic RV pacing has led to the development of pacemaker algorithms designed to minimize RV pacing when activation of the ventricles can be achieved through the native His-Purkinje conduction system.

TABLE 12.1. Pacemaker nomenclature

Position	1	2	3	4	5
	Chamber paced	Chamber sensed	Response to sensing	Rate regulation	Multisite pacing
	O = None	O = None	O = None	O = None	O = None
	A = Atrium	A = Atrium	T = Triggered	R = Rate Response	A = Atrium
	V = Ventricle	V = Ventricle	I = Inhibit		V = Ventricle
	D = Dual (A + V)	D = Dual (A + V)	D = Dual (T + I)		D = Dual (A + V)

Most frequently used programs are DDD, VVI, VDD, and DDI. Adapted from Bernstein et al., Pacing and Clinical Electrophysiology 2002[14]

References

1. Zheng ZJ, Croft JB, Giles WH, Mensah GA. Sudden cardiac death in the United States, 1989 to 1998. *Circulation.* Oct 30 2001;104(18):2158 2163.

2. Rosamond W, Flegal K, Furie K, et al. Heart disease and stroke statistics – 2008 update: a report from the American Heart Association Statistics Committee and Stroke Statistics Subcommittee. *Circulation.* Jan 29 2008;117(1).e25–e146.

3. Preliminary report: effect of encainide and flecainide on mortality in a randomized trial of arrhythmia suppression after myocardial infarction. The Cardiac Arrhythmia Suppression Trial (CAST) Investigators. *N Engl J Med.* Aug 10 1989; 321(6):406–412.

4. Julian DG, Camm AJ, Frangin G, et al. Randomised trial of effect of amiodarone on mortality in patients with left-ventricular dysfunction after recent myocardial infarction: EMIAT. European Myocardial Infarct Amiodarone Trial Investigators. *Lancet.* Mar 8 1997;349(9053): 667–674.

5. Moss AJ, Zareba W, Hall WJ, et al. Prophylactic implantation of a defibrillator in patients with myocardial infarction and reduced ejection fraction. *N Engl J Med.* Mar 21 2002;346(12):877–883.

6. Bardy GH, Lee KL, Mark DB, et al. Amiodarone or an implantable cardioverter-defibrillator for congestive heart failure. *N Engl J Med.* Jan 20 2005;352(3):225–237.

7. Zipes DP, Camm AJ, Borggrefe M, et al. ACC/AHA/ESC 2006 guidelines for management of patients with ventricular arrhythmias and the prevention of sudden cardiac death – executive summary: A report of the American College of Cardiology/American Heart Association Task Force and the European Society of Cardiology Committee for Practice Guidelines (Writing Committee to Develop Guidelines for Management of Patients with Ventricular Arrhythmias and the Prevention of Sudden Cardiac Death) Developed in collaboration with the European Heart Rhythm Association and the Heart Rhythm Society. *Eur Heart J.* Sep 2006;27(17):2099–2140.

8. Blumenthal RS, Epstein AE, Kerber RE. Cardiovascular Disease and Commercial Motor Vehicle Driver Safety, FMCS, 2007

9. Epstein AE, Baessler CA, Curtis AB, et al. Addendum to "Personal and Public Safety Issues Related to Arrhythmias That May Affect Consciousness: Implications for Regulation and Physician Recommendations. A medical/ scientific statement from the American Heart Association and the North American Society of Pacing and Electrophysiology". Public safety issues in patients with implantable defibrillators. A Scientific statement from the American Heart Association and the Heart Rhythm Society. *Heart Rhythm.* Mar 2007;4(3):386–393.

10. Bristow MR, Saxon LA, Boehmer J, et al. Cardiac-resynchronization therapy with or without an implantable defibrillator in advanced chronic heart failure. *N Engl J Med.* May 20 2004;350(21):2140–2150.

11. Cleland JG, Daubert JC, Erdmann E, et al. The effect of cardiac resynchronization on morbidity and mortality in heart failure. *N Engl J Med.* Apr 14 2005;352(15):1539–1549.

12. Hunt SA, Abraham WT, Chin MH, et al. ACC/AHA 2005 Guideline Update for the Diagnosis and Management of Chronic Heart Failure in the Adult: a report of the American College of Cardiology/American Heart Association Task Force on Practice Guidelines (Writing Committee to Update the 2001 Guidelines for the Evaluation and Management of Heart Failure): developed in collaboration with the American College of Chest Physicians and the International Society for Heart and Lung Transplantation: endorsed by the Heart Rhythm Society. *Circulation.* Sep 20 2005;112(12):e154–e235.
13. Moss AJ, Brown MW, Cannom DS, et al. Multicenter automatic defibrillator implantation trial-cardiac resynchronization therapy (MADIT-CRT): design and clinical protocol. *Ann Noninvasive Electrocardiol.* Oct 2005;10(4 Suppl):34–43.
14. Bernstein AD, Daubert JC, Fletcher RD, et al. The revised NASPE/BPEG generic code for antibradycardia, adaptive-rate, and multisite pacing. North American Society of Pacing and Electrophysiology/British Pacing and Electrophysiology Group. *Pacing Clin Electrophysiol.* Feb 2002;25(2):260–264.
15. Wilkoff BL, Cook JR, Epstein AE, et al. Dual-chamber pacing or ventricular backup pacing in patients with an implantable defibrillator: the Dual Chamber and VVI Implantable Defibrillator (DAVID) Trial. *JAMA.* Dec 25 2002;288(24):3115–3123.

Chapter 13
Management of Acute Decompensated Heart Failure

Joseph M. Delehanty

Heart failure is one of the most commonly encountered diagnoses in patients admitted to the hospital in the United States. It is estimated that there are more than 1 million patients yearly who are discharged from the hospital with the diagnosis of CHF and this number is likely to rise dramatically with the aging of the population. The impact of an admission for CHF is tremendous. The mortality for all patients admitted with this diagnosis has been found to be ~ 4.0%[1] with subgroups of patients whose mortality is >20%. There is also a very high likelihood that such patients will be readmitted for the same diagnosis within the six months following discharge. The estimated cost of caring for these patients exceeds $14 billion. As heart failure is one of the most important diagnoses in hospitalized patients, it is essential that patients with heart failure be rapidly identified and treatment begun promptly.

IDENTIFYING THE HEART FAILURE PATIENT
Heart failure is a clinical diagnosis that is characterized by a number of clinical findings including volume overload, manifest by edema, neck vein distension, ascites and pulmonary congestion among other findings. In addition to the findings of volume overload, there may also be signs of impaired cardiac output such as cool and underperfused extremities, mental confusion, and cyanosis. In its most advanced form, it is very easy to identify the patient with moist rales, a third heart sound, edema, cool extremities,

J.D. Bisognano et al. (eds.), *Manual of Heart Failure Management*,
DOI: 10.1007/978-1-84882-185-9_13, © Springer-Verlag London Limited 2009

etc., as having heart failure. In practice, however, this kind of presentation is the exception rather than the norm. Many studies have shown that patient with chronic CHF may have extremely elevated cardiac filling pressures in the absence of findings of edema, rales on auscultation of the lungs and pulmonary congestion on chest X-ray. In spite of the variability of physical exam findings in patients presenting with CHF, symptoms of dyspnea and/or fatigue are almost universal, and CHF should be considered in the initial differential of most patients with such complaints and should prompt clinicians to look for additional clinical risk factors for CHF. Commonly encountered clinical comorbidities in patients with CHF include a history of hypertension, coronary artery disease, and diabetes. These conditions are encountered in 73%, 57%, and 44% of patients, respectively,[2] in a registry of CHF patients. Patients presenting with dyspnea and risk factors should be carefully examined for the signs of heart failure with careful ausculation to detect gallup rhythms and close examination of the jugular venous waveform. In addition to the history and physical exam, many have come to rely on laboratory testing and imaging to make the diagnosis of CHF. Certainly the presence of significant LV dysfunction in the correct clinical setting suggests the diagnosis of heart failure but it is being increasing realized that many patients hospitalized with CHF have relatively preserved LV function. In several series, 22–45% of patients with the diagnosis of CHF had preserved LV ejection fractions.[2,3] This percentage is likely to increase in coming years as more patients with hypertension age and develop findings of what has been referred to as diastolic dysfunction or heart failure with preserved LV function. All patients presenting with heart failure should have a measurement made of ejection fraction done if one has not been done recently. In addition to being useful in some situations for the diagnosis of CHF, it is also important to distinguish patients with preserved LV function from those with impaired LV function. Although much of the acute treatment in these two groups is similar, the long-term treatment strategies for managing patients with preserved LV function differs significantly for the strategy used in patients with LV dysfunction.

Many clinicians have come to rely on the measurement of biomarkers, specifically B-type natriuretic peptide levels, to make the diagnosis of heart failure. In the correct clinical setting, elevation of plasma BNP (or nt-pro-BNP) levels certainly helps to confirm the diagnosis and the diagnosis of CHF should be questioned in individuals with low BNP levels (<50–100).[4] It should be mentioned that BNP levels can be elevated in other conditions that produce dyspnea such as acute myocardial infarction and pulmonary embolism and that one should not rely on a single lab test determination to make the diagnosis of CHF.

RISK STRATIFICATION OF THE HEART FAILURE PATIENT

Once the diagnosis of heart failure has been made in the acute setting, it is important to try and ascertain the severity of heart failure as this will to a large extent determine the course of therapy that is needed for the patient. A simple algorithm has been devised using data immediately available on presentation to determine risk of mortality.[1] It uses the BUN, systolic blood pressure, and creatinine to divide patients into low (<5% mortality), intermediate (>5<13% mortality), and high (>13% mortality) with those patients with a BUN < 43 mg/dl, SBP > 115 mmHg, and creatinine <2.75 mg/dl being low risk and those patients without each of these criteria falling into the highest risk category and likely requiring more intensive therapy.

Another approach that has been found to be useful is to divide patients into categories based on either their measured or estimated hemodynamic profiles.[5] Specifically, this involves using the presence or absence of congestion and the adequacy of perfusion. Those patients who have evidence of congestion, manifest by the presence of edema, ascites, neck vein distention, orthopnea, etc. would be considered as being "wet and warm" if they did not have signs of inadequate perfusion such as cool extremities, hyponatremia, poor renal function, narrow pulse pressure etc. Congested patients with such findings would be considered as "cold and wet." Those patients without signs of congestion but with impaired perfusion would be considered as "cold and dry" and finally those without congestion and without impaired perfusion would be considered "warm and dry." The "warm and dry" category refers primarily to those patients who are well compensated and will not be discussed here. Although somewhat of an oversimplification, this strategy allows one to concentrate on treatment of the specific hemodynamic abnormality in each patient as will be discussed later.

CAUSES OF DECOMPENSATION

The majority of patients presenting with decompensated heart failure have a preexisting diagnosis of heart failure, and it is important to try and determine the reason for the acute decompensation. Common reasons for decompensation include medication and dietary non-compliance, and it is important to try and obtain history regarding both medication use as well as diet. One should also ask about nonprescription drug use as many NSAIDs are available in nonprescription form and can result in significant sodium retention in the patient with CHF. In the patient with ischemic heart disease, it is essential that ischemia be excluded as a cause of decompensation as management of the ischemia will be an essential part of the treatment plan. It should be mentioned that one must use caution in using the troponin level alone to diagnose ischemia in this population, as it has been well demonstrated that troponin can be elevated in the patient with advanced heart failure in the absence of coronary artery disease or myocardial infarction.[6] Atrial fibrillation is a common occurrence in the patient with CHF and may result in acute deterioration particularly if the rate is uncontrolled. Other arrhythmias such as ventricular tachycardia and heart block are much less commonly encountered as causes of decompensation. Other medical conditions may also result in deterioration of a previously stable heart failure patient, particularly infections and this should be excluded, particularly in the elderly patient who may not present with the typical signs and symptoms of infection.

Although many patients present rather acutely, it has been shown that admission for CHF is often preceded by a period of weight gain in the week prior to admission[7] raising the question of whether earlier intervention may be able to prevent the admission.

INITIAL MANAGEMENT OF ACUTE DECOMPENSATED HEART FAILURE

In contrast to the state of chronic heart failure which can be viewed as predominantly a neurohumoral disorder, acute decompensated heart failure can be viewed primarily as a hemodynamic disorder, and therefore interventions should be directed at the primary hemodynamic abnormalities. The majority of patients presenting will fall into the category of "wet and warm" and in this population, the interventions should be aimed at reducing the congested state. In such patients presenting with significant respiratory distress as a result of pulmonary edema, this will require that the respiratory status is stabilized as quickly as possible. Some patients may require intubation as a result of respiratory failure. In many such patients, however, noninvasive mechanical ventilation with BIPAP is very helpful and can avert intubation.[8] The positive pressure provided by such ventilation not only improves ventilation but also provides some degree of preload and afterload reduction, improving the central hemodynamics of the patient in heart failure. It is worth attempting this form of ventilation before endotracheal intubation in most patients as it may allow time for additional therapy aimed at treating the pulmonary congestion.

In those patients presenting with the "wet and warm" profile, the cornerstone of treatment will be diuretic and vasodilator therapy. It is important to institute prompt diuretic therapy at an appropriate dosage. Many of these patients will have been taking high doses of oral diuretics as an outpatient, and in these cases, it is usual to start with at least the equivalent dose given in intravenous form. We have frequently been using continuous infusions of furosemide with good effect. A bolus dose of half of the usual outpatient dose followed by an infusion of between 5 and 20 mg/h is frequently used with good effect. Although there is little data on the superiority of the infusion compared with intravenous bolus dosing, we find that it allows better titration of the diuretic response in many cases. The patient who does not respond to initial intravenous diuretic therapy may require the addition of a thiazide diuretic such as Diuril, HCTZ, or metolazone to augment the response. It is important to frequently assess the response to initial diuretic therapy allowing for rapid escalation of dose in those paients who are not responding to initial therapy. Renal doses of dopamine have also been used in this setting, although these data to support this are not overwhelming.

The diuretic response to this regimen may be dramatic, and it is important to follow serum electrolytes closely to monitor the development of hypokalemia and/or metabolic alkalosis. This can usually be managed with aggressive potassium repletion but occasionally it is useful to add a potassium sparing diuretic such as amiloride or spironolactone. Spironolactone plays a role in the chronic management of systolic heart failure and should be the preferable agent is such cases. Extreme metabolic alkalosis will occasionally require the addition of the carbonic anhydrase inhibitor acetazolamide (Diamox). There is some evidence that ultrafiltration can be used effectively in such situations rather than diuretic therapy.[9] This requires specialized resources and is not currently widely available. The amount of fluid to be removed in such patients is variable. Many patients present with significant volume overload of 5–10 L. The usual practice is to remove as much fluid as needed to normalize cardiac filling pressures. Assessment of filling pressures without the use of hemodynamic monitoring can be difficult, however. Assessment of neck vein distention can be helpful and in those patients with an elevated JVP, normalization of the venous pressure is a reasonable goal. Some have advocated the use of serial measurement of plasma BNP levels as a guide to adequacy of therapy.[10] Another approach is to push diuretic therapy until there are objective signs of diminished cardiac output such as hypotension and/or worsening renal function.

Acute administration of potent vasodilating agents such as intravenous nitroprusside and nitroglycerine can be used with good effect in the patient with advanced, decompensated heart failure. The patient who presents with acute heart failure in the setting of severe hypertension is usually very responsive to vasodilator therapy. In spite of presenting with an impressive degree of pulmonary congestion, such patients may not be significantly volume overloaded, and it is not unusual to have these patients become somewhat hypotensive after being given diuretics and vasodilators and it may be necessary to give fluid after control of the hypertension. The use of nitroprusside requires careful monitoring and is probably best accomplished in the setting of hemodynamic monitoring.

Nesiritide is a human recombinant form of B-type natriuretic peptide that has vasodilating and natriuretic property, and has been shown to produce hemodynamic benefit in the acute heart failure population. It is an expensive agent and has not shown clear-cut clinical benefit and should probably be used in select patients with CHF and not as first-line therapy for acute decompensated heart failure.

Another issue that frequently arises is the concomitant use of chronic medications particularly ACE-I and β-blockers. We would recommend that unless there is significant azotemia or hypotension, that ACE-I be continued whenever possible.

β-blocker therapy is now considered standard for patients with chronic heart failure and one commonly encounters patients with chronic heart failure on β-blocker therapy who are admitted with decompensation. In some cases, the decompensation can be directly traced to the initiation of therapy with β-blockers or with an increase in the dose. In these situations, the drugs should obviously be stopped or the dose reduced. This is a relatively rare occurrence, however, and it is more frequent to see patients who have been stable on a dose of β-blocker who then present with decompensation presumably unrelated to the use of these agents. In patients presenting with the "wet and warm" profile, β-blockers should be continued at their usual dose unless hypotension occurs. In those patients in whom it is thought that impaired cardiac output is playing a role, it is often prudent to either hold the β-blocker or reduce the dose. Once patients have achieved their target in terms of volume removal, they can be transitioned to oral diuretics and doses of vasodilators and β-blockers can be maximized. One should be cautious about trying too hard to titrate these agents in the early stages of treatment as the ability to achieve fluid removal may be impaired by hypotension.

The patient who presents with the "cold and wet" profile poses significant challenges in terms of therapy. While fluid overload is a major component of the clinical presentation, diuresis alone is unlikely to be successful unless concomitant interventions directed at improving cardiac output are also employed. This usually means the administration of inotropic agents and/or intravenous vasodilators. Vasodilator use may be limited by low blood pressure in this very ill group of patients. The most commonly used inotropic agents are the synthetic β-agonist Dobutamine and the phosphodiesterase inhibitor Milrinone. Both agents increase contractility in the myocyte by increasing intracellular cAMP levels. Dobutamine stimulates adenylate cyclase and CAMP production and milrinone prevents breakdown of cAMP. Both drugs have been used successfully in this setting. Milrinone has more vasodilating properties and has the potential advantage of being more potent than Dobutamine in the presence of β-blockers. It should be mentioned that there are no studies that have demonstrated a survival benefit to the use of inotropic agents in decompensated heart failure but many clinicians have found them to be very useful in the management of the most severe cases. In those individuals who have responded favorably to a course of inotropic therapy, oral vasodilators should be titrated up as the drugs are being weaned. There is a small group of patients who deteriorate with the removal of inotropic therapy, and such patients might be considered for chronic inotropic therapy.[11]

Some have advocated the use of invasive hemodynamic monitoring to guide treatment of patients with decompensated heart failure with the goal of therapy being normalization of hemodynamic parameters as much as possible. A randomized trial of this approach compared with standard therapy without the use of hemodynamic monitoring did not show any significant clinical benefit[12]; however, many clinicians do use hemodynamic monitoring to guide therapy, particularly in the sicker patients or those who are not responding to therapy in the expected fashion.

The "cold and dry" profile patient also presents many challenges. It is important to be sure that there is not occult volume overload as fluid administration in this setting will prove to be detrimental. This is one setting where the use of a pulmonary artery catheter may be beneficial in determining the volume status of the patient. In patients in whom volume depletion is confirmed, judicious volume administration will be helpful and after that has been accomplished careful attempts to uptitrate the ACE-I and β-blockers can be attempted.

A minority of patients presenting with decompensated heart failure will not respond to aggressive treatment and exhibit signs of progressive heart failure. Many of these patients will develop what has been referred to as a "Cardiorenal Syndrome" characterized by progressive azotemia and renal dysfunction. This may respond at least temporarily to initiation of inotropic support but may persist and require stopping beneficial but potentially nephrotoxic agents such as ACE-I and ARBs. The combination of oral hydralazine and nitrates can be used instead of ACE-I/ARB in this situation. The development of the cardiorenal syndrome is an ominous finding and many would advocate escalation of therapy at the first signs of it with mechanical circulatory support and/or urgent transplantation in patients who are deemed to be candidates for such therapy. Patients who are not candidates for such interventions will often progress to a terminal condition and need to be considered for a more palliative approach.

The patient who responds to acute therapy can then be transitioned to aggressive chronic therapy using standard therapy with ACE-I/ARB, β-blockers, diuretics, digoxin, and aldosterone antagonists. In the sicker patients, particularly those with the "cold and wet" profile, titration of beta-blockers needs to be done slowly as there is a real risk that the patient could deteriorate if the dose is escalated too quickly. Those patients with systolic dysfunction and a bundle branch block pattern on ECG may be candidates for biventricular pacing. Such procedures should only be done once the patient has stabililized and is tolerating an outpatient regimen. Experience with placing biventricular pacemakers in patients who are actively decompensated has been very discouraging and should be avoided.

It has been well documented that the risk for readmission following discharge is very high in this population. A number of strategies have been employed to reduce the risk of readmission. The most successful have used an aggressive home-based intervention strategy with close monitoring of weight, dietary habits, concomitant medication use, and frequent outpatient follow up encounters.[13] In addition to being effective in preventing readmission in heart failure patients, such instructions are now considered quality measures and need to be documented in all patients discharged with the diagnosis of heart failure.

CONCLUSION

Decompensated heart failure is a major cause of mortality and morbidity in the United States and the rest of the world. In addition to accounting for over 1 million hospitalizations, it accounts

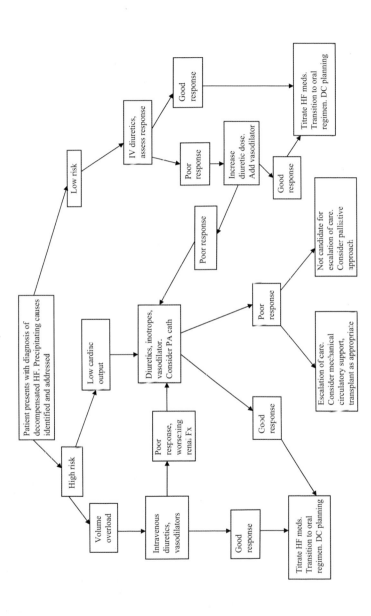

FIGURE 13.1.   High risk features include abnormal vital signs, hypoxia, BUN > 43, Creatinine > 2.75, multiple heart failure admission, acute changes on ECG.

for a large percentage of the current health care expenditures and the likelihood is that this will increase dramatically over the coming years as the population ages. In spite of the rather diverse manner in which decompensated heart failure can present, most patients can be identified early. Once identified as having decompensated heart failure the pathophysiology can usually be identified and specific therapy aimed at the primary pathophysiologic process can be instituted. Figure 13.1 is a flow diagram that is useful in the evaluation and management of hospitalized patients. Although there have been advances in the acute management of hospitalized patients with heart failure, there is still much to be done to reduce the likelihood of readmission in the months following discharge as well as in prevention of the hospitalization.

References

1. Fonarow GC, Adams KF, Abraham WT, Yancy CW, Boscardin WJ. Risk stratification for in-hospital mortality in acutely decompensated heart failure. JAMA 2005;572–80.
2. Adams KF, Fonarow GC, Emerman CL et al. Characteristics and outcomes of patients hospitalized for heart failure in the United States: Rationale, design and preliminary observations from the first 100,000 cases in the Acute Decompensated Heart Failure National Registry (ADHERE). Am Heart J 2005;149:209–16.
3. Cleland JCG, Swedberg K, Follath F et al. The Euroheart survey programme: A survey of the quality of care among patients with heart failure in Europe. Eur Heart J 2003; 24:442–63.
4. Maisel AS, Krishnaswamy P, Nowak RM et al. Rapid measure of B-type natriuretic peptide in the emergency diagnosis of heart failure. N Engl J Med 2002;347:161–7.
5. Grady KL, Dracup K, Kennedy G et al. Team management of patients with heart failure: A statement for healthcare professionals from the Cardiovascular Nursing Council of the American Heart Association. Circulation 2000; 102:2443–56.
6. Horwich TB, Patel J, MacLellan WR, Fonarow GC. Cardiac troponin I is associated with impaired hemodynamics, progressive left ventricular dysfunction, and increased mortality rates in advanced heart failure. Circulation 2003; 108:833–8.
7. Chaudhry SI, Wang Y, Concato J, Gill TM, Krumholz HM. Patterns of weight change preceding hospitalization for heart failure. Circulation 2007; 116:1549–4.
8. Antonelli M, Conti G, Rocco M et al. A comparison of non-invasive positive pressure ventilation and conventional mechanical ventilation in patients with acute respiratory failure. N Engl J Med 1998; 339: 429–35.
9. Costanza MR, Guglin ME,Saltzberg MT et al. Ultrafiltration versus intravenous diuretics for patients hospitalized with acute decompensated heart failure. J Am Coll Card 2007; 49:675–83.

10. Kazanegra R, Cheng V, Garcia A et al. A rapid test for B-type natriu-
    retic peptide correlates with falling wedge pressures in patients treated
    for decompensated heart failure: A pilot study. J Cardiac Fail 2001;
    7:21–9.
11. Hershberger RE, Nauman D, Walker TL, Dutton D, Burgess D. Care
    processes and clinical outcomes of continuous outpatient support with
    inotropes (COSI) in patients with refractory end stage heart failure.
    J Cardiac Fail 2003; 9:180–7.
12. The ESCAPE investigators. Evaluation study of congestive heart failure
    and pulmonary artery catheterization effectiveness. JAMA 2005;294:
    1625–33
13. Stewart S, Horowitz JD. Home based intervention in congestive heart
    failure: Long-term implications on readmission and survival.
    Circulation 2002;105:2861–6

Chapter 14
Heart Failure Clinics:
A Strategy for Success

Mary Beth Earley

INDICATIONS FOR A HEART FAILURE CLINIC

The physical, emotional, and financial burden of heart failure (HF) on our society is incontrovertible.An estimated 5.3 million Americans carry the diagnosis, with 80% of the men and 70% of the women under the age of 65 dying within 8 years.[8] In 2008, we will pay an estimated $31.7 billion in direct health care fees, while facing a substantial indirect cost of more than $3 billion linked to lost productivity resulting from the morbidity and mortality associated with HF syndrome.[13] The scientific and medical communities continue to research a plethora of new drugs, devices, and surgical techniques designed to combat the widespread fallout of this devastating disease.

Interestingly, one of the more important recent findings has nothing to do with new medical or surgical therapies. Granger et al. discovered that the morbidity and mortality benefits in the CHARM trial were evident for both candesartan *and* placebo groups if patients adhered to taking > 80% of their prescribed pills,[7] suggesting that improvement in HF outcomes depends on patients' abilities to care for themselves. Unfortunately, a significant barrier to a patient becoming an effective self-manager is our current health care system itself.

Inherent to our present health care system's culture is a focus on the identification and treatment of acute illness. A patient can be triaged, diagnosed, and treated shortly after presentation to a local

J.D. Bisognano et al. (eds.), *Manual of Heart Failure Management,*
DOI: 10.1007/978-1-84882-185-9_14, © Springer-Verlag London Limited 2009

emergency room or urgent care center; however, the patient's role throughout the process remains largely passive. In direct contrast, successful management of people with chronic disease states such as HF requires active patient participation in concert with a truly interested health care team.[16–17] One way of accomplishing this is through the development of a multidisciplinary HF clinic that focuses not only on providing cutting-edge evidenced-based medical and surgical HF therapies, but also on providing the comprehensive education and counseling that lays the foundation for effective patient self-management and adherence to a treatment plan.[9]

POTENTIAL BARRIERS

There are many potential barriers to developing a successful HF clinic. Administrative support, space, and resources all need to be well-defined ahead of time, while regional reimbursement issues must be addressed. For example, Medicare fee-for-service may not pay for certain things such as nutritional counseling or medication education for a patient; however, a nutritionist or pharmacologist could be asked to speak at a regularly scheduled support group meeting. More frequent clinic visits may be indicated if telemonitoring and home care are not covered. Additional challenges such as building a broad referral base and establishing productive associations with expert specialty groups (such as electrophysiologists and cardiac surgeons) are dependent not only on the clinical expertise of the providers, but on their communication skills as well. The medical director and staff must be able to sell the concept of the HF clinic to other providers within the community.

HEART FAILURE CLINIC DESIGN

Numerous descriptions of HF clinics can be found throughout the literature.[1–2,5,10–12,14] There are accounts of physician-led programs, nurse-run programs, team-managed programs, and programs such as ours that are a combination of two or more of these designs (Figure 14.1). No matter what the structural design of the clinic, it appears that the key to success, which can be defined in terms of reduction in hospitalizations, emergency room visits, and healthcare costs along with improved event-free survival, lies in good chronic disease management and that good chronic disease management consists minimally of early outpatient visits after discharge, frequent follow-up evaluations, and patient education that focuses on self-management.[3–4,6,15,18]

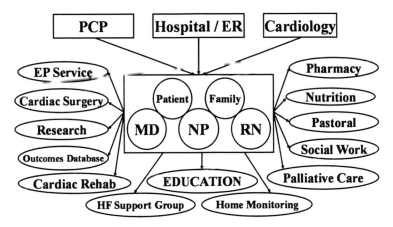

FIGURE 14.1. Heart failure clinic.

ESSENTIAL ELEMENTS OF A HEART FAILURE CLINIC

Just as an ACE-inhibitor and beta-blocker are the foundation of HF medical therapy, the successful HF clinic requires two crucial building blocks as well. The first is an educated, engaged patient that becomes an involved health care partner, and the second is a well-organized health care team armed with protocol-driven algorithms based in the latest clinical evidence. This alliance results in productive interactions and improved outcomes in HF management.[16–17]

The Educated Patient

It is important not to confuse patient education with patient self-management. Simply handing information to patients will not make them effective self-managers. Early in the professional relationship (and periodically throughout), practitioners must assess each patient's individual needs, concerns, values, beliefs, preferences, goals, and lifestyle. This knowledge helps identify what may motivate a patient and what barriers to effective self-management may exist. An awareness of a patient's baseline understanding of the disease process, level of literacy, cognitive abilities, and psychological state as well as their access to social and financial resources will help the team provide individualized education and treatment plans specifically tailored to each patient's needs. Additional strategies that we have found useful to increase a patient's awareness and involvement include:

- Provide educational materials in multiple formats including print, electronic, and video.
- Although all require education, focus on those patients with class III and IV as their risk of associated morbidity and mortality is significantly higher.
- Be clear on all expectations and explain their importance. Provide learning tools that summarize the critical points and expectations that can be referred back to quickly and often (Figure 14.2).
- Write everything down for the patient - who to call, when to call, changes in medications, follow up appointments, when to go for labs, and so on.
- Utilize every resource at your disposal to target specific needs and behaviors. Build a multidisciplinary team that can address both the pharmacological *and* nonpharmacological aspects of HF care. This team may include social work, pastoral care, financial counselor, translator, palliative care, cardiac rehab, nutrition, cardiac surgery, electrophysiology services, pharmacy, and home health services.
- Offer regular support group meetings. If a clinic cannot afford to have a nutritionist, PharmD or psychiatrist on staff, ask one to volunteer an hour of their time and come speak at the support group.
- Prepare them on what to expect. Let them know that they might feel worse temporarily while increasing their beta-blocker.
- Have frank discussions early on (and periodically thereafter) about the risk of sudden cardiac death, advanced directives, and end-of-life care. Describe the continuum of HF therapy including polypharmacy, ICDs and biventricular pacemakers, surgical therapies, ventricular assist devices, and transplant.
- Be accessible 24/7 with a dedicated team interested in chronic disease management.
- Be responsive. Call back promptly and coordinate tests and procedures smoothly.
- Push patients until they push back. Encourage better diet, medication up-titration, and more physical activity.
- Do not give up. What does not work today may work tomorrow, particularly in the case of medication up-titration. Discourage discontinuing a drug with life-lengthening benefits at the first sign of side effects and try again the next month.
- Repeat. Repeat. Repeat.

The Proficient Healthcare Team
In effective clinics, experienced practitioners rapidly assess a patient's clinical status and self-management skills, and then tailor

SYMPTOMS YOU MAY NOTICE	REASONS TO CALL YOUR DOCTOR/NURSE	WEIGHT	DIET / FLUIDS	MEDICATIONS	ACTIVITY
▼ Excessive weakness and fatigue. ▼ Shortness of breath, especially when lying down. ▼ A dry, hacking cough. ▼ Bloating in stomach, with a decreased appetite and nausea. ▼ Swelling in the feet and ankles.	▼ Your weight increases 2-3 pounds overnight or 5 pounds in a week. ▼ Increased shortness of breath that is unusual for you while resting, during the night, or with activity. It is not normal for you to need to sit in an upright position (such as in a recliner or propped on several pillows) to sleep at night. ▼ If you notice unusual swelling in your hands, face, lower legs, feet, ankles or abdomen -OR- f you notice a "full feeling" in your stomach and have less appetite or nausea.	▼ Weigh yourself every morning after you first get out of bed, after going to the bathroom and before eating or drinking anything. ▼ Weigh yourself in the same amount of clothing, without shoes, and on the same scale. The scale should be on a hard, flat surface.	▼ Take the saltshaker off the table. ▼ Limit your salt (sodium) intake to <2000 mg a day. ▼ Avoid hi-salt items: -canned soup/bouillon -canned vegetables -cold cuts/deli meats -ham/bacon/cheese -hot dogs/sausages -tomato juice -prepackaged meals -soy sauce Read the labels!	▼ Know your medications: -how much -how often -what it's for -side effects ▼ Take your medications exactly as prescribed and carry a list of them with you at all times. ▼ Do NOT skip medication. Do not stop TAKING them without talking with your health care provider.	▼ A little activity can make you feel a lot better. ▼ Go for a walk, visit a friend, or perhaps do some gardening. ▼ Wait at least one hour after meals. Avoid extreme temps. ▼ Stop and rest if you feel tired or short of breath.
FOLLOW-UP APPOINTMENTS ▼ Make sure you follow-up with your family doctor and your heart doctor within a few weeks after you are discharged. Call for appointments if not arranged for you at the time of discharge.	▼ If you notice persistent dizziness, blurred vision, headache, unsteadiness, extreme fatigue or a racing heartbeat. ▼ Weight gain. ▼ Decreased urination. ▼ **If you have unrelieved chest pain, unrelieved shortness of breath, confusion or fainting: Call 9-1-1 immediately.**	▼ Record your weights on the back of this form and compare it to the last 4 or 5 readings. ▼ A rapid weight gain may be a sign your body is retaining fluid and may indicate a need for a change in your treatment plan.	▼ Season with lemon and herbs for flavor. "Mrs. Dash and Molly McButter" recipe club: 1-800-622-3274 www.mrsdash.com www.mollymcbutter.com ▼ Eat lean meats, whole grains, fresh fruits and vegetables. ▼ Limit your TOTAL fluid intake to 2 liters (or 2 quarts) a day. ▼ Avoid alcohol.	▼ If you miss a dose, do not "double up" on your next dose. ▼ Check with your health care provider before taking any over-the-counter remedies.	**SMOKING** ▼ Nicotine makes your heart work harder. **STOP!** ▼ Avoid second-hand smoke. ▼ "QUIT LINE" 1-866-NY-QUITS (1-866-697-8487)

FIGURE 14.2. Patient teaching tool.

their medical management according to evidenced-based protocols and guidelines. The resulting collaboration between the
patient and the provider team leads to effective problem solving
and the creation of an individualized long-term plan with mutually
advantageous goals. The plan of care should call for consistent,
regular, and often frequent follow-up. Payors should find that the
relatively low costs of close monitoring and frequent clinic visits
will decrease the rate of costly hospitalizations and testing.

Once the plan of care is agreed upon by the practitioner and
the patient, the next most important step is *communication* of that
plan. Communication with the primary care physician (PCP), the
primary cardiologist, and with any specialist that the patient may
have, such as an endocrinologist or rheumatologist, is essential.
All notes should be dictated and sent out as quickly as possible.
Once a patient's HF therapy has been fully optimized (both pharmacological and non-pharmacological aspects) and the patient
has demonstrated stability on that therapy, the patient may choose
to follow up with just his PCP and/or cardiologist. Additional
strategies we have found useful for creating proficient healthcare
teams include:

- Look for a dedicated medical director (MD) who is interested in
  HF management and understands the huge benefits that can be
  achieved from the available treatments. The MD needs to be an
  excellent communicator; someone who can sell his vision to the
  referring physician base within the community.
- Set up an advanced practice nurse or physician assistant who
  is experienced in the care of HF patients to guide patients and
  manage other nursing and office staff in their interactions with
  the patients. This person should be familiar with the applicable
  ICD codes and be able to bill either independently or "incident to."
- Develop a multidisciplinary team to address the many complex
  issues that surround chronically ill patients. Again, this team may
  include social work, pastoral care, financial counselor, translator,
  palliative care, cardiac rehab, nutrition, cardiac surgery, electrophysiology services, pharmacy, and home health services.
- Follow established research-based protocols and guidelines.
- Anticipate a minimum of ½ hour for each patient follow-up visit
  with daily appointments available for urgent visits, particularly
  on Mondays and Fridays.
- Have office staff "prep" patient charts right before their visit,
  confirming that it is current with the most recent visit note, corre-
  spondence, lab work and test results, and those copies have been
  forwarded to the PCP, cardiologist, and consulting physicians
  as well.

- Assess the patient's understanding of disease and treatment plan at each visit, while looking for adherence concerns.
- Screen patients on a "HF Continuum"
  - Perform a comprehensive history and physical examination. Document NYHA functional class and AHA/ACC stage at each visit.
  - Review all medications, both prescribed and over-the-counter.
  - Routine HF testing, including labs, ECG, echo, functional status, and arrhythmia screening.
  - Hunt for any reversible causes of HF.
  - Conduct specialized testing, which may include stress and viability testing, cardiac MRI, echocardiogram, coronary angiography, and right heart catheterization.
  - Expect that the benefits of medical therapy may take months to become evident; always keep options such as transplant and destination ventricular assist device therapy in mind – both yours and the patient's – when appropriate.
  - Refer in a timely fashion for testing, implantable defibrillators, resynchronization therapy, cardiac surgery, ventricular assist device and transplant evaluation, palliative care and hospice.
  - Streamline the treatment plan from the start with such things as once a day dosing regimens for simplicity, generic medications to save money, standing lab orders for convenience, appointment times that minimally interrupt work schedules or family life, short waiting room times and parking validation to encourage frequent follow-up, and so on. Adherence is more likely with collaboration, communication and a clear course of action.

CONCLUSION

HF clinics employing chronic disease management strategies have been shown to reduce the rate of hospitalizations, emergency room visits, and overall healthcare costs while improving event-free survival.[3–4,6,15,18] Although larger and more longitudinally designed studies are needed, a multidisciplinary HF clinic that focuses not only on providing cutting-edge evidenced-based medical and surgical HF therapies, but also on providing the comprehensive education and counseling can lay the foundation for effective patient self-management and adherence to a treatment plan.[9]

References

1. Advocate Health Care (2003) Advocate's disease management program reduces readmissions for CHF and asthma. Perform Improv Advis; 7:44–47
2. Albert NM, Young JB (2001) Heart failure disease management: a team approach. Cleve Clin J Med; 68:53–62; discussion 63–64

3. Akosah K, Schaper AM, Havlik P, Barnhart S, Devine S (2002) Improving care for patients with chronic heart failure: The importance of a disease management program. Chest; 122:906–912

4. Cline CMJ, Israelsson BYA, Willenheimer RB, et al. (1998) Cost effective management program for heart failure reduces hospitalization. Heart; 80:442–446

5. Dahl J, Penque S (2000) The effects of an advanced practice nurse-directed heart failure program. Nurse Pract; 25:61–62, 65–68, 71–74

6. Fonarow GC, Stevenson LW, Walden JA (1997) Impact of a comprehensive heart failure management program on hospitalization readmission and functional status of patients with advanced heart failure. J Am Coll Cardiol; 30:725–732

7. Granger BB, Swedberg K, Ekman I, et al. (2005) Adherence to candesartan and placebo and outcomes in chronic heart failure in the CHARM program: double-blind, randomized, controlled clinical trial. Lancet; 366:2005–2011

8. Heart Disease and Stroke Statistics — 2008 Update, American Heart Association

9. Heart Failure Society of America, Executive summary (2006) HFSA 2006 Comprehensive Heart Failure Practice Guideline. J Card Fail; 12:10–38

10. Henrick A (2001) Cost-effective outpatient management of persons with heart failure. Prog Cardiovasc Nurs; 16:50–56

11. Katon W, Von Korff M, Lin E, Simon G (2001) Rethinking practitioner roles in chronic illness: the specialist, primary care physician, and the practice nurse. Gen Hosp Psychiatry; 23:138–144

12. McAlister FA, Steward S, Ferrua S, McMurray JJJ (2004) Multidisciplinary strategies for the management of heart failure patients at high risk for readmission. A systematic review of randomized trials. J Am Coll Cardiol; 44:810–819

13. National Heart, Lung, and Blood Institute. Fact Book, Fiscal Year 2006. With all estimates by Thomas Thom of NHLBI

14. Paul S (2000) Impact of nurse-managed heart failure clinic: a pilot study. Am J Crit Care; 9:140–146

15. Ramahi T, Longo MD, Rohlfs K, et al. (2000) Effect of heart failure program on cardiovascular drug utilization and dosage in patients with chronic heart failure. Clin Cardiol; 23:909–914

16. Wagner EH, Austin BT, Davis C, Hindmarsh M, Schaefer J, Bonomi A (2001) Improving chronic illness care: translating evidence into action. Health Aff.(Millwood); 20:64–78

17. Wagner EH, Bennett SM, Austin BT, Greene SM, Schaefer JK, Vonkorff M (2005) Finding common ground: patient-centeredness and evidence-based chronic illness care. J Altern Complement Med; 11:Suppl 1, S7–S15

18. Whellan DJ, Gaulden L, Gattis WA, et al (2001) The benefit of implementing a heart failure disease management program. Arch Intern Med; 161: 2223–2228

Chapter 15
Patient Self-Management Strategies for Heart Failure

Anna E. Lambert and Jill R. Quinn

INTRODUCTION

Heart failure (HF) is a condition that is a result of disease progression that is extremely complex and can be difficult to medically manage. HF patients and families are expected to be able to monitor themselves for changing symptoms and make lifestyle changes to prevent worsening HF. Self-care management presents a significant challenge to patients with HF who present to our clinics, offices, and hospitals in varying degrees of HF. Educating and motivating patients and families to follow established guidelines for self-care management is paramount to the goal of minimizing the progression of the condition and maintaining the best quality of life and reduced hospitalizations. We must integrate education and promote self motivation for behaviors that will optimize their HF treatments and regimens prescribed for them.

KEY TOPICS FOR PATIENT SELF MANAGEMENT

There are three broad topics of patient education that are of relevant importance in the management of patients with HF at all stages. They are lifestyle changes, medications, and knowing when to seek advice. Providing education and ensuring comprehension of these three areas has the greatest chance of success in delaying the progression of the HF process and reducing unnecessary hospital admissions.

J.D. Bisognano et al. (eds.), *Manual of Heart Failure Management*,
DOI: 10.1007/978-1-84882-185-9_15, © Springer-Verlag London Limited 2009

Lifestyle Changes

Lifestyle changes are probably the most difficult area for the patient and their families to adapt to and maintain success. There are often relapses in behaviors as described by various adult learning principles accepted today. These principles will be discussed later in the chapter.

Heart Healthy Diet

Components of a heart healthy diet include low fat, low cholesterol, low sodium, and reduced calories appropriate for weight control. The patient newly diagnosed with HF will require education on food label reading. Label reading education should have emphasis on serving size, calorie content, fat, and sodium content. The provider may begin with an assessment of how food choices are made in the household. The person responsible for shopping and cooking, as well as the patient consuming the diet should be included in education. Utilization of available nutrition experts such as dieticians is useful in the interdisciplinary team effort of education for HF. Emphasis on sodium awareness is one of the most important aspects of the Heart Healthy Diet (?ref) education for the HF patient. A familiar cycle to most practitioners is the dynamic balance between level of sodium restriction and diuretic dosing. The inpatient generally follows the sodium restriction as hospital meals are delivered to them. Once the patient is discharged however, unless the patient or person preparing meal selections are competent in reading labels for sodium content, there is often a period of necessary diuretic titration that needs to occur. The high sodium content of most convenience foods is often surprising to most patients that are not familiar with reading labels. Titration of diuretics necessitates communication with the provider. Failure to maintain some level of surveillance by the provider often results in readmissions. A follow-up phone call program which contacts the patient at specific intervals may be helpful in preventing readmissions due to over or under diuresis.

Smoking Cessation

Smoking as well as any consumption of nicotine such as chewing tobacco contributes to heart disease. Nicotine addiction is a powerful entity that even the most well-meaning patient will have difficulty overcoming. Various mechanisms to assist the patient in achieving cessation are available today. These include medications such as varenicline – a nicotine receptor blocker, nicotine replacement patches, and lesser known and accepted therapies such as hypnosis and acupuncture. Smoking cessation requires some level of behavior modification, which is discussed further in following sections on adult learning principles.

Weight Control and Exercise

This is a challenging area particularly for the HF patient. Regular exercise is an important part of weight control for healthy patients; however, exercise tolerance may be a significant deterrent for the advanced HF patient. Those with New York Heart Association (NYHA) class III or class IV HF are limited by their physical ability to engage in meaningful exercise. Inquiry into the patient's level of comfort with stair climbing is often a good indication of their exercise tolerance. The six minute walk test is another simple measure to gauge the level of activity tolerance. Even advanced stage HF patients should be encouraged to commit to regular walking on flat surfaces. Local malls are an excellent safe location to enable patients to walk in a controlled environment.

Weight control is a complicated paradigm for the HF patient as it is also affected by degrees of fluid retention. The patient's dry weight is the measure that should be compared with optimal body mass index (BMI), for a tailored approach to an appropriate calorie control and exercise plan. The concept of fluid retention and the effect on weight must be understood by the patient in order for them to be successful in true weight control. Weight loss due to diuresis is not true weight loss, and unless the patient understands this concept, they may not be successful in achieving optimal BMI. In the very advanced HF patient, cardiac cachexia may necessitate nutritional supplements for optimal health.

Alcohol Moderation

Excessive alcohol intake can be associated with alcohol induced cardiomyopathy. Alcohol consumption by the HF patient should be minimal if at all. Evidence based literature is limited in supporting amounts of alcohol intake. The caloric contribution as well as any contraindications related to medications should be considered in the recommendation for any particular patient.

Medications

The HF patient is faced with the prospect of taking multiple daily medication combinations to control the progression of remodeling in HF. These include antihypertensive medications, angiotensin converting enzyme inhibitors (ACEi), diuretics, anti-lipidemic agents, beta blockers, angiotensin release blockers (ARB), insulin, aspirin, anti-arrhythmic, and inotropic agents. The patient can be easily overwhelmed by the number of medications prescribed for them, not to mention the common side effects and cost of prescription drugs today, and have difficulty with medication compliance. People expect to feel better after taking a medication as commonly experienced with the sudden improvement in symptoms after taking a few antibiotic doses. However, many of the medications prescribed for HF patients often cause side effects that cause the patient to feel worse before feeling better. One example is initiation of ACEis. This paradox is common as the medication is titrated to therapeutic range. This is a particular challenge to the health care team who must keep the confidence of the patient during this critical period.[1] Medication review and reinforcement as well as encouragement to take all medications are important at every patient encounter. There are often many changes that occur between dosing, addition of medications, or holding doses. The process of medication reconciliation is a valuable process for both the provider and the patient as all medications are validated for both. The opportunity for clarification and education is prime during the practice of comparing lists.

Knowing When to Seek Advice

One of the early goals of patient education is to assure the comprehension of which symptoms are important enough to have follow-up either by a phone call or visit to the office or clinic. The symptoms related to worsening HF generally include symptoms related to weight gain, change in breathing, or intolerance to activity. Table 15.1 stratifies symptoms actions to take for the exhibited symptom.

It is important that patients feel comfortable to call the office for any complaints, and receive positive reinforcement for follow-up. A reluctance to call may result in an inpatient admission, where it could have been avoided with simple early intervention.

KEYS TO SUCCESS

Providing patient education either in person or as in handing out a booklet is not enough to promote lifestyle changes that are necessary for sustained healthy behaviors. Education is one facet of the complete cycle of behavioral change. Merely having knowledge about an issue does not necessarily motivate humans to change behavior. A complete assessment of the patients' readiness to accept new information as well as their preferred learning style, and identification of any barriers are the basis of achieving desired compliance. There are many theoretical models to describe and guide the process of change. Many have been developed and studied in relationship to smoking cessation, prevention of sexually transmitted diseases,[2] and promoting diet and exercise routines.

TABLE 15.1. The "Heart Failure Symptom Awareness and Action Plan". The first column represents the symptcm severity indicated by color code escalating from green to red (most serious). The second column represents the action recommended based on the symptom category

STRONG ✷ HEALTH
STRONG MEMORIAL HOSPITAL

HEART FAILURE SYMPTOM AWARENESS AND ACTION PLAN

SMH 1638

SYMPTOM		ACTION
If you have: • No shortness of breath • A usual amount of ankle swelling • No weight gain • No chest pain • No change in your usual activity level	➡	Your symptoms are under control. • Continue taking your medications as ordered • Continue to weigh yourself everyday • Follow a low-salt diet • Keep all physician appointments
If you have any of the following: • Weight gain of 3 or more pounds • Increased cough • Increased swelling • Increased shortness of breath with activity • Increased number of pillows needed to sleep	➡	You may need an adjustment of your medications. Call your health care contact for instructions: Name: _____ Phone Number: _____
If you have any of the following: • Shortness of breath at rest • Wheezing or chest tightness at rest • Need to sit in chair to sleep • Weight change of more than 5 pounds over or under normal weight • Dizziness, extreme fatigue, or falling	➡	You need to see a doctor now. Call your doctor now: Name: _____ Phone Number: _____
If you have: • Unrelieved shortness of breath • Unrelieved chest pain • Confusion or fainting	➡	**Call 9-1-1 Immediately**

Rev 5/07

Elements of Adult Learning Theories

1. Knowles (1980) Adult Learning Principles[3, 4]
   a. Adults learn best when topic content builds upon previously understood material.
   b. Active participation between the patient and caregiver facilitates learning, as opposed to lecturing.
   c. Adults need to practice and reinforce new skills – reading labels.
   d. Adults need reinforcement – following healthy diet and exercise regimes actually make the patient feel better.
   e. An opportunity to validate comprehension of a topic, or uncover any misconceptions increases learning.

2. Transtheoretical Model of Change[5] – The transtheoretical model is the most widely used models to assess readiness for and promote behavioral change. It is characterized by a nonlinear progression through the stages with expected occurrences of relapse before succeeding.
   a Precontemplation – no awareness of the need to change.
   b. Contemplation – information gathering and consideration of change.
   c. Preparation-internalizing the need to change behavior and planning steps to make a change
   d. Action – implementing practices or actions of the desired behavior.
   e. Maintenance – incorporating the new behavior into the normal pattern of living.
   f. Termination – the undesired behavior has been eliminated.

3. Blooms Taxonomy[6] – There are three components to learning:
   a. Knowledge (Cognitive)
   b. Attitude (Emotional)
   c. Skills (Psychomotor)

4. Kubler – Ross[7] Stages of Grief

A diagnosis of "heart failure" can be frightening and has no cure. Only palliative treatments can be provided in many cases. The patient may progress through the stages of grief when presented with such a new diagnosis, with interpretations of anticipatory loss of health and life.

a. Denial
b. Anger
c. Bargaining
d. Depression
e. Acceptance

The models and principles of learning as noted above each bring relevant and important aspects to the patient diagnosed with HF. Our patients present to us in various stages of HF as well as in different stages of acceptance of their diagnosis, and motivation to attain the best level of health possible given the progression of disease.

It certainly takes an interdisciplinary team (primary care physician, HF cardiologist, nurses, cardiac rehab staff, nutritionist, pharmacist, exercise physiologist, social worker, and pt. family) to motivate and change the behaviors of the HF patient. It is not only the patient themselves that is incorporated into counseling, but also their significant others must be included for sustained success. Teaching, learning, motivation, and resultant change is a cyclical process that is often heralded by occasional relapses before self-efficacy[8] is attained. In the case of the HF patient, this is complicated by the progressive nature of the disease process.

Motivation: Strategies to Motivate
The patients' readiness to change is a measure of their motivation. Human beings need a reason to change. They are most open to information and motivation to change, after a life threatening event. There may be a logical conclusion linking lifestyle and an acute event during the immediate period following the event. In less obvious circumstances, data may be helpful to positively or negatively reinforce behaviors. Data may include blood pressure recordings, weight measurements, or a journal of subjective feelings. Quantitative elements can be compared with activities of the patient whether that is diet, exercise, or medication compliance. If the patient themselves can make the connection of the relationships between these factors, the more motivated they may remain. Self-efficacy or the belief that they are capable to continue desired behaviors including compliance with diet, medication, and exercise regimes is the goal. Coaches, mentors, and support persons or groups are adjunctive measures to reinforce and support the patient toward autonomous control of their lifestyle and medical regime compliance. Occasional relapse into undesirable behaviors should be expected as a natural process of change.

A complete assessment of the patient must include evaluations of: the emotional state, current level of knowledge of the disease process, stage of readiness to learn, preferred learning style, and prevalence of any barriers.

Identification of Barriers

Cognitive Changes Associated with HF

Recent studies have demonstrated that progressive HF may also result in cognitive decline.[9],[10] This may impact the patients' ability to completely process the information that is presented to them. It is recommended that significant others are included in all instruction and dialogue. Repetition and the opportunity to validate information promote learning. Formal assessment of the patient's cognitive level can be determined by neuro-cognitive testing. Informal assessments can be done by administering simple tests such as the Mini Mental State Examination.[11]

Patients with cognitive challenges may need creative tools to assist them in their compliance. Many versions of pill boxes are available from simple plastic cases with the days of the week printed on them, to sophisticated electronic reminders. This type of patient may require structure in the form of written reminders, journals etc. Secondary causes of neurological change should also be acutely evaluated.

Cost

Medical costs are exceedingly complex and must be considered within the comprehensive scope of care. An evaluation of the insurance coverage and knowledge of the nuances of the patient's insurance coverage may be determining factors of selections of treatments. It makes no sense to prescribe medications that the patient may never be able to afford and therefore comply with. There are programs available from the drug companies for patients that meet certain financial need criteria. This may be an option for some. Generally, pharmacists and social workers have the most up to date information about such programs.

Perceived Value

Generally speaking HF patients have more than just a few medications prescribed. There are often side effects and adjustment periods of titrations associated with the drugs. The patient must be counseled relative to the risk/benefit balance of the drug. They are more likely to adhere to the prescribed regime if they understand the risk benefit equation.[12]

Depression

Depression is a common finding in the HF patient[9] and must be considered and treated for optimal success in promoting self management. Depression may be the result of several components related to progressive heart disease, such as overall declining health, activity intolerance, dependence on medications and devices, burden on family and finance, and consideration of their own mortality.

Lack of Support from Family

Involving family members in education and counseling is vitally important; however, lack of support is indeed a barrier. Lifestyles among and between family members of the same household are usually consistent. If smoking is a desired lifestyle change but other family members continue to engage in the behavior, then intuitively the less likely the patient will be successful in smoking cessation. Biological family members of the HF patient are genetically linked, and may in fact share risk factors known and those yet uncovered. This presents an excellent topic for discussion and potentially a motivating factor for the family members. The social worker is a valuable team member to assist in the comprehensive assessment of the patients support network.

TOOLS AND TECHNOLOGIES

Two essential items for the HF patient are a symptom awareness chart and a mechanism to record daily symptoms and numerical data. The symptom awareness chart is a necessary component to guide the patient regarding when they should escalate care. Early intervention for symptoms may prevent the need for a hospital admission.

Education of Relevance of Symptoms

Tools such as those found in Table 15.1 include a simple color coded document that grades symptoms and guides the patient to the appropriate level of care that they should seek. Early intervention for weight gain related to fluid overload may make the difference between early treatment and escalation of failure. There are numerous tools available on the internet from reliable sources, by searching the term HF.

Self-Monitoring

A reliable mechanism to record weight, activity, vital signs, and symptoms is helpful in promoting self-efficacy. Tools can be as simple as paper and pencil or ready made documents and electronic programs. Computer savvy patients may collect and document their information onto spreadsheets. The emphasis is on *self* monitoring, which contributes to real-time feedback to the patient. Self-monitoring must also be linked with the knowledge of when to report findings.

Remote Monitoring

Telehealth is a growing field that is readily applicable to the care of the HF patient. Telehealth consists of transfer of patient data to a provider electronically. There are devices available today that are able to transmit weight, blood pressure, and heart rate in addition to logging of symptoms. The information is reviewed by practitioners. Reimbursement, however, does vary according to insurance coverage. Telehealth is thought to be an area of tremendous potential growth.

Support Groups

Community or Hospital Based Support Groups are helpful for the patient and family in multiple ways. The concept of support groups is a well-accepted entity. Sharing of similar feelings, experiences, ideas, and hope are some of the benefits of participation in a support group. Knowing that they are not alone in the situation is valuable to patients (Table 15.2).

RESOURCES

SUMMARY

Strategies to optimize patient self management in HF are dependent upon assessing the patient's readiness to accept change, and customizing the approach to education, and follow-up care. There are many elements to achieving self efficacy for the HF patient. These are chiefly related to the patients understanding of the disease process, the stage of acceptance of their current level of health, and the resources available to them. HF patients require individualized assessment of both physical and emotional health with customized care planning to achieve and maintain the highest level of self management possible. The provider must also understand that the process toward self management is not linear.

TABLE 15.2. The "Daily Weight and Symptom Chart". The column headings indicate date, weight, presence of shortness of breath, number of pillows used for sleep, presence of cough, and presence of swelling including location. There is an additional column for comments or questions. The patient is instructed to complete the chart daily and bring it with them to any appointments

DAILY WEIGHT & SYMPTOM CHART

Instructions:
1. Use the same scales each day. Be sure the scales are on a flat, hard surface.
2. Weigh each morning after urinating, but before eating breakfast. Wear similar weight clothing each time you weigh yourself.
3. Check any symptoms that you may have on the chart below.
4. Notify your doctor if you gain 3 pounds in one day, or 5 pounds in a week.
5. Bring this form and your medication bottles with you *every* time you visit the clinic or hospital!

DATE	WEIGHT	SHORT OR BREATH (Yes/No)	NUMBER OF PILLOWS FOR SLEEP	COUGH (Yes/No)	SWELLING (Where?)	COMMENTS/QUESTIONS

References

1. Williams, GC, Rodin, GC, Ryan, RM, et al. (1998) Autonomous Regulation and Long-term Medication Adherence in Adult Outpatients. Health Psychology 17:269–76.
2. Denison J (1996) Behavior Change – A Summary of Four Major Theories. The AIDS Control and Prevention Project, implemented by Family Health International.
3. Knowles MS (1980) The Modern Practice of Adult Education: From Pedagogy to Andragogy. Cambridge University Press; New York: 43–44.
4. Conklin J (1995) Principles of Adult Learning: How Can They Help. New Jersey Nurse. 25(7):7.
5. Prochaska JO, Velicer WF (1997) The Transtheoretical Model of Health Behaviour Change. American Journal of Health Promotion 12:38–48.
6. Dickson VV, McMahon JP (2008) Optimal Patient Education and Counseling. Cardiac Nursing: A Companion to Braunwald's Heart Disease. Saunders, St Louis.
7. Kubler-Ross Model at http://en.wikipedia.org/wiki/K%C3%BCbler-Ross_model, retrieved from the www December 15, 2007.
8. Bandura A (1997) Self-Efficacy: The Exercise of Control. WH Freeman and Company, New York.
9. Romanelli J (2003) Depression and Neuro-cognitive deficits are common comorbid conditions in ambulatory heart failure patients. The Journal of Heart and Lung Transplantation (22) 1.
10. Sangha SS, Uber PA, Park MH, et al. (2002). Difficult Cases in Heart Failure: The Challenge of Neurocognitive Dysfunction in Severe Heart Failure. Journal of Congestive Heart Failure 8:232–234.
11. Kurlowicz L, Wallace, M. (1999). The Mini Mental State Examination. The Hartford Institute for Geriatric Nursing.
12. Carrick, R, Mitchell, A, Powell, RA, et al. (2004). The Quest for Well Being: A Qualitative Study of the Experience of Taking Antipsychotic Medication. Journal of Psychology Psychotherapy 77:19–33.

Chapter 16
Nutrition Interventions in Heart Failure

Bethany Barney and G. Ronald Beck

The benefits of pharmacological treatments for heart failure (HF) have been well documented in multiple studies. Nonpharmacological treatments such as nutrition therapy are becoming more widely recognized as important factors in the prevention and treatment of HF. Traditional HF nutrition therapy has primarily focused on dietary sodium and fluid restrictions. In addition to these commonly prescribed restrictions, other items such as micronutrient supplementation are emerging as potential areas for further study into their role in the treatment of HF. Thorough patient education and follow-up evaluation is essential to encourage a patient's compliance with prescribed dietary recommendations. Studies have shown that including a registered dietitian on a multidisciplinary team can have a positive effect on dietary compliance and lead to reduced hospital admissions and their associated costs.[1] Because patients' needs change as their HF progresses, nutrition therapy should be individualized according to a patient's particular requirements. For those at risk of developing HF (ACC/AHA stages A and B), nutrition therapy is aimed at managing general cardiovascular risk factors and comorbidities such as hypertension, dyslipidemia, obesity, and diabetes. In patients with diagnosed HF (ACC/AHA stages C and D), the focus is on controlling symptoms and maintaining quality of life, meeting elevated nutritional requirements, and preventing acute decompensations and hospitalizations.[2]

J.D. Bisognano et al. (eds.), *Manual of Heart Failure Management*,
DOI: 10.1007/978-1-84882-185-9_16, © Springer-Verlag London Limited 2009

ACC/AHA STAGES A AND B: REDUCING THE RISK FOR CARDIOVASCULAR DISEASE AND DEVELOPING HF

Although no specific nutritional recommendations exist for the prevention and treatment of HF, the American Heart Association (AHA) Diet and Lifestyle Recommendations provide general guidelines for reducing the risk of developing cardiovascular disease. The guidelines are designed to be flexible and encourage healthy lifestyle modifications. Table 16.1 summarizes the AHA 2006 Diet and Lifestyle Recommendations and provides practical tips for their implementation.

The AHA also makes recommendations for dietary supplements shown to reduce cardiovascular disease risk.

Fish Oil Supplements

According to the AHA, fish oil supplements are appropriate in those individuals with documented coronary artery disease at a dosage of 1 g/day. Patients with hypertriglyceridemia may also benefit from fish oil supplements at an increased dosage of 2–4 g/day.[3]

Plant Stanols/Sterols

Plant stanols and sterols are naturally occurring substances found in plant cell membranes that are chemically similar to animal cholesterol. These substances compete with cholesterol in the gastrointestinal tract to decrease cholesterol absorption. Consumption of plant stanols and sterols at levels up to 2 g/day as part of healthy diet has been shown to lower LDL cholesterol levels up to 15% without lowering HDL.[4] Plant stanols and sterols can be found in small quantities in many fruits, vegetables, nuts, seeds, legumes and grains; however, in order to reach therapeutic amounts, most consumers need to include foods in their diet that have been supplemented with plant sterols and stanols. These substances have been added to a wide variety of foods, including certain margarines, beverages such as orange juice, and some yogurt products. Stanols and sterols can also be found in capsule form. These items need to be consumed consistently each day to have a positive effect on cholesterol levels.

ACC/AHA STAGE C

The above recommendations continue to apply to patients classified as ACC/AHA stage C, those with left ventricular dysfunction with current or prior HF symptoms. In addition, these patients may need to pay close attention to sodium and fluid intake to help manage symptoms.

TABLE 16.1. 2006 AHA diet and lifestyle recommendations for cardiovascular disease risk reduction and practical tips for their implementation

AHA 2006 diet and lifestyle recommendation	Practical hints for implementation
Balance calorie intake and physical activity to achieve or maintain a healthy weight	Be aware of your caloric needs and the caloric content of food and beverages consumed. Include regular physical activity to help maintain caloric balance
Consume a diet rich in fruits and vegetables	Aim for a wide variety of fruits and vegetables, prepared with little or no added salt, sugar, and fat. Choose whole fruits and vegetables over juices for increased dietary fiber
Choose whole grain, high fiber foods	At least one-half of grain intake should come from whole grains. Foods rich in soluble fiber (commonly found in oats, beans, peas, barley, citrus fruits, strawberries, apples, and pears) have been shown to aid in lowering LDL cholesterol
Consume fish, especially oily fish, at least twice a week	Fish, particularly oily fish such as salmon, mackerel, lake trout, herring, sardines, and albacore tuna are rich in the omega-3 polyunsaturated fatty acids eicosapentaenoic acid (EPA) and docosahexaenoic acid (DHA). These have been shown to reduce the risk of sudden death and death from coronary artery disease
Limit your intake of saturated and *trans* fat and cholesterol	Aim for less than 7% of total calorie intake from saturated fat, less than 1% of calorie intake from *trans* fats, and less than 300 mg of cholesterol per day (less than 200 mg of cholesterol per day for those with heart disease). Choose lean meats and low fat dairy products in place of higher fat varieties

(continued)

TABLE 16.1. (continued)

AHA 2006 diet and lifestyle recommendation	Practical hints for implementation
Minimize your intake of beverages and foods with added sugars	Foods and beverages with added sugars contribute to total daily caloric intake without adding additional nutrients
Choose and prepare foods with little or no salt	The AHA recommends a reduction in sodium intake to 2,300 mg/day (limit to 2,000 mg/day for those with HF). Read food labels to compare foods and choose those lowest in salt. Do not add salt in cooking and reduce intake of highly processed, convenience foods that are high in salt
If you consume alcohol, do so in moderation	Patients with HF should avoid alcohol. However, those patients who do drink alcohol should limit their daily intake: women, to no more than one serving, and men, to no more than two
When you eat foods that are prepared outside of the home, follow the AHA 2006 diet and lifestyle recommendations	Many foods prepared away from home contain added salt, sugar, saturated and *trans* fats and are low in fiber. Carefully choose items that fit into the AHA Diet and Lifestyle Guidelines

Adapted from Lichtenstein et al.[3].

Sodium and Fluid Balance

Although no concrete evidence exists to quantify a specific recommendation for sodium restriction in HF, the general consensus is that patients should limit their daily sodium intake to 2,000 mg/day.[5] The first step in reducing sodium intake is often eliminating added salt both at the table and in cooking. Highly processed foods such as canned soups and vegetables, frozen dinners, convenience and other restaurant meals, processed meats and cheeses, and many condiments also contribute a large portion of sodium to the diet. Patients need to learn about reading labels and restaurant menus to assess the sodium content of the foods they eat. Patients with persistent volume overload despite following a low sodium diet and appropriate diuretic therapy may also need a fluid restriction, typically less than 2 L/day.[5] Those with hyponatremia may also require a fluid restriction.

Collaborative patient education regarding sodium and fluid restriction should occur on an ongoing basis to encourage compliance. One study investigated the impact of detailed dietary counseling by a registered dietitian compared to the standard care of providing only written education materials to patients. In this study, those patients who had individualized nutrition assessment, education, and follow-up evaluation by a registered dietitian had a significant reduction in daily sodium intake, while those who received literature without verbal instruction did not show a significant change in sodium intake.[6]

ACC/AHA STAGE D

Patients classified as ACC/AHA stage D, those with refractory, end-stage HF, often require individualized dietary intervention and management to address their specific issues. In these patients, factors such as decreased appetite, fatigue, early satiety, malabsorption, lack of variety on restricted diets, and emotional factors such as depression can have a negative impact on nutritional status. In addition, the hyperinflammatory, catabolic state often seen in advanced HF can further exacerbate nutrient imbalance leading to cardiac cachexia. Small, frequent meals are often best tolerated in those with malabsorption and early satiety. Strict dietary restrictions may need to be liberalized in patients with poor intake. Those who are not able to meet their nutritional needs may require oral supplements and enteral or parenteral support to improve their nutritional status. Detailed nutrition assessment and follow-up evaluation by a registered dietitian can help address these complex factors and may improve outcomes.

Calories
Studies have demonstrated that energy expenditure is increased in HF. Traditional daily recommendations of 25 kcal/kg for healthy adults and 30 kcal/kg for nutritionally depleted individuals may not be adequate in HF patients and could lead to weight loss. Normally nourished, clinically stable heart failure patients require a minimum of 28.1 kcal/kg/day. Nutritionally depleted and underweight patients require at least 31.8 kcal/kg/day to maintain body mass and counteract the effects of hypermetabolism. Hypocaloric diets for overweight and obese patients need to be used with caution, as they may lead to loss of lean body mass in patients who are catabolic.[7] Indirect calorimetry would be beneficial to help determine caloric goals in individual patients.

Protein
Clinically stable, normally nourished HF patients require a daily intake of at least 1.12 g of protein/kg to prevent negative nitrogen balance and counteract the effects of hypercatabolism. Those patients who are nutritionally depleted require higher levels of protein, at least 1.37 g/kg/day.[7]

MICRONUTRIENT SUPPLEMENTATION
There is growing evidence that there is a relationship between micronutrient deficiencies and HF. Micronutrients can be linked to HF in various ways, through their impact on myocyte energy production, their effect on calcium homeostasis, or their regulation of oxidative stress.

Vitamins and Minerals

B Vitamins
The B vitamins are water soluble and stored in only small amounts in body tissues. They require consistent consumption to maintain adequate stores. Thiamine acts as a coenzyme in carbohydrate metabolism. Deficiencies can cause impaired oxidative metabolism and a build up of pyruvate and lactate, resulting in vasodilation.[8] This vasodilation can lead to high output HF and a reduced ejection fraction. The reported prevalence of thiamine deficiency in HF ranges from 3 to 96% depending on a patient's nutritional status and supplement use, variations in their medication regimes, and differing methods used to measure the patient's thiamine stores.[9] A number of factors commonly seen in HF may lead to thiamine deficiencies: poor intake, restricted diets that may limit foods high in thiamine, and increased urinary losses of thiamine

in patients on diuretics. Supplementation with thiamine has been examined in several small studies. One study provided HF patients on long-term furosemide therapy (less than or equal to 80 mg/day for a minimum of 3 months) with a dose of 100 mg intravenous thiamine twice daily for 6 weeks. These patients showed a significant improvement of left ventricular ejection fraction.[9]

Folate and vitamin B_{12} have received some attention in heart disease because of their correlation with homocysteine levels. An elevated homocysteine level is a risk factor for cardiovascular disease because of its impact on oxidative damage and its negative effect on vascular endothelium. Folate is responsible for converting homocysteine into methionine with vitamin B_{12} acting as a cofactor. Thus, supplementation of folate and vitamin B_{12} in deficient patients may aid in lowering homocysteine levels.[8]

Riboflavin (vitamin B_2) and pyridoxine (vitamin B_6) play a role in energy production and are essential to the formation of red blood cells. Vitamin B_6 is also involved in the metabolism of homocysteine. A deficiency in vitamin B_6 is a risk factor for coronary heart disease and carotid artery disease, likely related to resultant elevated homocysteine levels.[8] There has been little investigation into the connection between vitamin B_2 and vitamin B_6 deficiencies and HF.

Additional research needs to be conducted that further examines the relationship between B vitamin deficiencies and heart failure. Perhaps these studies will provide more specific guidance regarding methods for testing for deficiencies and dosages for repletion. Until that time, it may be prudent to recommend a supplement containing B vitamins to HF patients who are at risk for deficiencies.

Antioxidants: Vitamin C, Vitamin E, and Selenium

Patients with HF have increased levels of oxidative stress, which may be attenuated with supplementation of certain antioxidants. Vitamin C supplementation has been shown to lower blood pressure in hypertensive patients. It may also lead to improved endothelial function in diabetic patients and smokers, as well as in patients with endothelial dysfunction related to hypercholesterolemia.[8]

In middle-aged adults, a high vitamin E intake has been linked to a reduced occurrence of coronary heart disease. Decreased oxidative stress and decreased platelet aggregation is also seen with higher levels of vitamin E intake. Despite these findings, there are limited data to support the routine use of a vitamin E supplement in HF patients.[8]

Selenium deficiencies, although rare, have been linked to development of cardiomyopathy, ischemic heart disease, and peripheral vascular disease. A codeficiency in vitamin E may further exacerbate these conditions. There have been no studies that have solely examined selenium supplementation in HF.[8]

Calcium and Vitamin D

Calcium and vitamin D play many important roles in the functioning of the cardiovascular system. Calcium is important for proper muscle contraction and maintaining normal heart rhythms. Patients in the later stages of heart failure are prone to low calcium levels due to the urinary calcium losses with loop diuretics, poor dietary intake, and decreased absorption of calcium.

Vitamin D is emerging as a potential nonpharmacological therapy to help prevent and treat HF. Vitamin D has a positive impact on the cardiovascular system through its anti-inflammatory effects and its role in maintaining proper muscular function, lowering blood pressure and improving glucose tolerance. One study in men with HF showed that a 50 mcg daily supplement of cholecalciferol for 9 months suppressed the release of the proinflammatory cytokine tumor necrosis factor-alpha, a compound known to contribute to the development of HF. The study group also showed increased levels of the anti-inflammatory cytokine interleukin 10, which has cardioprotective effects. Both treatment and nontreatment groups showed improved left ventricular function; however, the change from baseline was not significantly different between study groups.[10] Other studies have been conducted using smaller dosages of vitamin D, with little or no effect on cytokine concentrations.[11] Heart failure patients may benefit from a calcium and vitamin D supplement, although additional research needs to be conducted to establish recommendations for dosages.

Magnesium

Magnesium depletion is common in HF patients because of the magnesium wasting effects of loop and thiazide diuretics. Low magnesium levels can lead to arrhythmias and other symptoms such as fatigue. Hypomagnesemia can also have a negative effect on sodium and potassium balance. Supplemental magnesium may help alleviate these symptoms.[8]

Coenzyme Q_{10} (Ubiquinone)

Coenzyme Q_{10} is a vitamin-like compound essential in mitochondrial production of adenosine triphosphate (ATP). It also acts as an antioxidant and has a stabilizing effect on cell membranes. Serum and myocardial coenzyme Q_{10} levels can be depleted in HF patients, with some studies reporting deficiencies in up to

50% of patients. Several studies have been conducted to examine the effects of coenzyme Q_{10} supplementation in HF. These have yielded mixed results. Some studies have demonstrated increased stroke volume and cardiac output in treatment groups. Others have resulted in increased exercise capacity, improved functional status and quality of life scores. Not all studies produced the same positive outcomes, but no negative effects were reported. Dosages of 50–150 mg/day, levels thought to be safe and well tolerated, were most commonly studied.[12]

Carnitine

Carnitine plays an important role in myocardial energy production. Up to 50% of HF patients may be deficient in carnitine. A handful of small studies have examined carnitine supplementation in HF patients, yielding some positive results. Participants showed improved exercise tolerance, reduced left ventricular dilation, and improved survival. Other studies did not yield the same results.[12] Additional research needs to be conducted to further examine the potential benefits of carnitine supplementation in HF patients.

Taurine

Taurine is an amino acid essential to the regulation of intracellular calcium. Studies have shown some HF patients to be deficient in taurine, perhaps related to the negative effect tumor necrosis factor-alpha has on the biosynthesis of taurine. Few studies have examined the effect of taurine supplementation in HF, although one study did result in improved hemodynamics and functional capacity in patients provided with supplemental taurine.[12]

Creatine

Creatine, a nitrogen-containing compound made in the body from amino acids, contributes to the production of ATP in skeletal muscle. One study showed a positive effect on skeletal muscle strength and endurance in HF patients provided with short-term oral creatine supplementation. There was no effect on ejection fraction, however.[8] The long-term safety and efficacy of creatine supplementation would need to be examined before routine use in HF patients can be recommended.

Combined Nutritional Supplementation

Due to the complex metabolic pathways involved in the pathogenesis of HF, it is unlikely that supplementation with a single nutrient will yield significant improvement in outcomes. One study examined the effect of multinutrient supplementation in patients with HF. The supplement included calcium, magnesium, zinc, copper, selenium, vitamin A, thiamine, riboflavin, vitamin B_6, folate, vitamin B_{12}, vitamin C, vitamin E, vitamin D, and coenzyme Q_{10}. After 9 months, the treatment group showed a 5% improvement in left ventricular ejection fraction and a significant decrease in left ventricular volume. In addition, there were modest improvements in quality of life scores within the treatment group.[12]

References

1. Chapman D, Torpy J (1997) Development of a heart failure center: a medical center and cardiology practice join forces to improve care and reduce costs. The American Journal of Managed Care 3:431–437

2. Ershow AG, Costello RB (2006) Dietary guidance in heart failure: a perspective on needs for prevention and management. Heart Failure Review 11:7–12

3. Lichtenstein AH, Appel LJ, Brands M, Carnethon M, Daniels S, Franch HA, Franklin B, Kris-Etherton P, Harris WS, Howard B, Karanja N, Lefevre M, Rudel L, Sacks F, Van Horn L, Wionston M, Wylie-Rosett J (2006) Diet and lifestyle recommendations revision 2006. A scientific statement from the American Heart Association Nutrition Committee. Circulation 114:82–96

4. Lichtenstein AH, Deckelbaum RJ for AHA Nutrition Committee (2001) Stanol/Sterol ester-containing foods and blood cholesterol levels. Circulation 103:1177–1179

5. Hunt SA, Abraham WT, Chin MH, Feldman AM, Francis GS, Ganiats TG, Jessup M, Konstam MA, Mancini DM, Michl K, Oates JA, Rahko PS, Silver MA, Stevenson LW, Yancy CW (2005) ACC/AHA 2005 Guideline update for the diagnosis and management of chronic heart failure in the adult: a report of the American College of Cardiology/ American Heart Association Task Force on Practice Guidelines (Writing Committee to Update the 2001 Guidelines for the Evaluation and Management of Heart Failure) American College of Cardiology Web Site. Available at http://www.acc.org/qualityandscience/clinical/guidelines/failure/update/index.pdf

6. Arcand JL, Brazel S, Joliffe C, Choleva M, Berkoff F, Allard JP, Newton GE (2005) Education by a dietitian in patients with heart failure results in improved adherence with a sodium-restricted diet: A randomized trial. American Heart Journal 150:716e1–716e5

7. Aquilani R, Opasich C, Verri M, Boschi F, Febo O, Pasini E, Pastoris O (2003) Is nutritional intake adequate in chronic heart failure patients? Journal of the American College of Cardiology 42:1218–1223

8. Witte KKA, Clark AL, Cleland JGF (2001) Chronic heart failure and micronutrients. Journal of the American College of Cardiology 37:1765–1774

9. Sica DA (2007) Loop diuretic therapy, thiamine balance, and heart failure. Congestive Heart Failure 13:244–247

10. Schleithoff SS, Zitterman A, Tenderich G, Berthold HK, Stehle P, Koerfer R (2006) Vitamin D supplementation improves cytokine profiles in patients with congestive heart failure: a double-blind, randomized, placebo-controlled trial. American Journal of Clinical Nutrition 83:754–759

11. Vieth R, Kimball S (2006) Vitamin D in congestive heart failure. American Journal of Clinical Nutrition 83:731–732

12. Allard JL, Jeejeebhoy KN, Sole MJ (2006) The management of conditioned nutritional requirements in heart failure. Heart Failure Review 11:75–82

Chapter 17
Psychological Considerations

Mark W. Nickels

Stress, anxiety, and depression can have significant impact on the heart by increasing the likelihood of developing cardiac problems and also worsening cardiac outcomes in patients who already have cardiac problems. Stress can give rise to arrhythmias.[1] Anger can lead to increased risk of coronary heart disease (CHD).[2–6] Thirty to fifty percent of patients with coronary artery disease (CAD) who experience mental stress can have transient symptomatic ischemia, left ventricular dysfunction, and even fatal arrhythmias.[7–9] Heart failure (HF) patients are at increased risk of MI following episodes of anger or anxiety.[10] In fact, psychological distress confers a greater risk for acute myocardial infarction (MI) than hypertension, obesity, or diabetes.[11]

In addition to the impact of stress and mood states on the heart, social factors also appear to play a role in cardiac difficulties. Social isolation and living alone increase the risk of recurrent coronary events in cardiac patients, and can lead to worse cardiac outcomes.[12] The fewer the number of support people available to HF patients, with whom they can discuss their problems, is a predictor of increased mortality at 1 year.[13] Limited social supports can have an indirect negative impact on cardiac outcomes. Living alone and having fewer supports point toward the possibility of poorer adherence to medical regimens, which in turn predicts worse cardiac outcomes.[14]

J.D. Bisognano et al. (eds.), *Manual of Heart Failure Management,*
DOI: 10.1007/978-1-84882-185-9_17, © Springer-Verlag London Limited 2009

A BI-DIRECTIONAL LINK
Patients with HF are more likely to develop depression or experience anxiety and psychosocial distress as a result of their heart disease. Further, living with HF challenges coping abilities, and can lead to diminished job function, worse stamina, changes in household roles/duties, and more social isolation. As a result, patients can experience a loss of control and increased frustration. These things can adversely impact cardiac function, and deepen the cycle of stress and cardiac dysfunction.

COPING WITH HF
Coping with serious medical problems typically occurs in stages. Shock and denial are often initially present, followed by sadness and anger, and then hopefully acceptance. However, HF patients are often faced with chronic health symptoms, a future of uncertainty and the fear of unending health threats. This can impede reaching a state of acceptance. Patients may find themselves in a typical cycle of enduring their symptoms until the emotions well up and pierce their efforts to manage and accept their illness. At that point they experience emotional suffering. The suffering then abates and patients endure once again until the next episode of suffering occurs. As health problems persist and gradually worsen, the periods of suffering typically increase in frequency and intensity. Patients with limited premorbid coping abilities will experience more frequent and intense episodes of emotional suffering. Suffering is often experienced as frustration, and over time, this can become chronic. It can be difficult to deal with chronic frustration. Patients often tend to either underexpress or overexpress it. For those who hold in their frustration, blow-ups can occur that are well out of proportion to the precipitating circumstance. For patients who overexpress frustration, there is ongoing irritation, often in the form of complaints and blaming. Over time, a sense of pessimism can evolve along with a passive stance toward health care and life. This is the breakdown of effective coping.

THE ROLE FOR HEART FAILURE CLINICIANS
Healthcare providers can help patients in their efforts to cope with both heart failure and the psychological issues associated with it. They can do so by acknowledging the reality of patients' health situations and then asking them about their feelings. The process of asking about, listening to, and then reflecting back the feelings being expressed is helpful in itself. This can help reduce the sense of vulnerability patients feel by enhancing the quality of the treatment relationship. Very commonly, the feelings being expressed by

these heart failure patients are normative. Because providers are in the position to see many such patients and see typical patterns of feelings and responses, they can tell patients it is usual to feel upset by declining physical abilities or to feel frustrated by the challenges of finding new ways to occupy their days. Such seemingly small comments can be helpful to both patients and families by normalizing the experience. In addition, such comments can go a long way in reducing a sense of inadequacy, fear, and "being in it alone." It can be difficult at times for providers to refrain from prematurely offering medical solutions to the feelings being expressed. However, when patients bring their feelings into the discussions, it can be beneficial to pursue these in some depth. In addition to the process of listening and exploring feelings, providers should also explain to patients what they can expect in the near future. It is helpful to include information about the heart, what patients might expect from medications, possible future symptoms, and typical psychosocial experiences. Such information, by virtue of its predictive value, can help reduce uncertainty and associated anxiety.

Keeping patients involved in their health care is very important. Exercise, to the degree possible, can be prescribed. Ongoing physical outlets not only help with general health, but also can help reduce frustration. Patients can be offered relaxation techniques and meditation exercises. These interventions can reduce perceived distress and for some can reduce catecholamine production, thereby reducing the physiological impact of stress on the heart.[1,15,16] Providers should ask patients to keep weight logs and track vital signs and other health parameters. Providers can ask patients to call the office periodically to check in, whether they are symptomatic or especially if they are not. For patients who have difficulties contacting the office or tracking their health care, clinicians should consider making regular phone calls to these patients to "check in" on them. This "open channel" for patients can help them feel less vulnerable, which in turn can reduce fear and its impact on symptom perception and unnecessary phone calls. Further, prescribing these things helps patients to become more proactive, counterbalancing tendencies toward passivity. Passivity can increase frustration. Hence, by reducing the degree of passivity, providers can help reduce patients' frustrations. Providers should highlight those things patients do well enough - whether it is self-tracking weights and vital signs, getting lab work done, finding useful outlets for feelings, or other helpful healthcare behaviors. This positive reinforcement can help patients feel a sense of competence. This in turn help provides hope and a degree of optimism – not necessarily for a cure or full return to function, but rather that they will be able to handle their health situations well enough. Optimism has been shown to have positive cardiac effects by decreasing the chance of CHD.[17]

Providers should routinely repeat directions several times and also give important directions in writing. Because of the relative hypoperfusion in HF patients, cognitive processing can be impaired, even in subtle ways, including memory and attention. These cognitive problems can contribute to adherence difficulties due to forgetfulness or reduced learning ability, which can then impact self-care through impaired symptom recognition and subsequent decision making.[18]

Clinicians can encourage patients to attend cardiac support groups. These groups often provide valuable information to patients and families, while offering connection with others in similar circumstances. This can be a potentially powerful counterbalance to a sense of isolation that can exist for some HF patients and families. In addition, the altruistic forces at work in group interactions are known to be one of the curative factors in groups.[19]

Psychotherapy and education in hospitalized patients with myocardial infarctions can reduce lengths of stay and the occurrence of CHF, lead to a faster return to normal activities, and have fewer symptoms of CAD even after 1 year.[20,21] As such, it appears that the use of counseling/therapy may have benefits into the future and could contribute to better long-term cardiac outcomes. Psychotherapy or counseling referrals should be considered in HF patients who have limited supports or who seem to have undue difficulty dealing with their heart disease. Working with a mental health professional can help patients acknowledge their health circumstances, deal with their feelings and frustrations, and help modulate the cycle of "enduring and suffering." Further, it can help mitigate undue excursions into thinking badly of one's self.

Finally, attention to family and loved ones can be of benefit, as a means of bolstering support systems. Similar to the patients, family members and loved ones must deal with role and duty changes because of the HF. They can develop frustrations and upsets with which they must cope, and need their own supports and protection against isolation. Providers can involve loved ones by asking them to come along with patients at the time of office visits, asking about their feelings, and then educating them about the normative experiences of families and friends who are dealing with HF patients. Referrals to support groups can be of value.[22]

DEPRESSION AND ANXIETY

Both depression and anxiety can increase the risk of CHD in a graded fashion.[23] There is ample evidence for the significant prevalence of depression in CHF patients – some studies indicate a nearly 50% prevalence.[24,25] Depression increases the risk of developing CHF in patients with risk factors for it,[26] and is a strong predictor of worsening HF in patients who already have CHF.[27] Depression can decrease adherence to medical regimens in cardiac patients,[28,29] further complicating health issues and contributing to distress. HF patients with depression are more likely to die from cardiac events or be medically rehospitalized, even when controlling for left ventricular ejection fraction and BNP levels.[30] Major depression can worsen cardiac outcomes,[24] and depression and social isolation increases mortality by 2.2–5.4 times over those without depression.[31]

Given this sobering data, it is important that HF providers monitor for depression, even if mild. This can be done through history-taking and the use of self-report instruments given to patients during office visits. Three such tools are the Patient Health Questionnaire or PHQ-9,[32] the Beck Depression Inventory or BDI,[33] and the Hamilton Rating Scale for Depression or HAM-D.[34] These well-validated instruments typically take little time and are easily used. Ongoing monitoring for depression is important even when depression is not present on initial exam. Depression can develop later in the course of heart problems. Havranek found an incidence of depression of 21% after the first year in patients that did not initially present with depression.[35]

If depression is present and mild, HF clinicians can take steps to help reduce symptoms. Problem-solving with patients - that is, working to engage them in how to address the cardiac, lifestyle, and their emotional needs – is not only a useful general approach but can help mood symptoms. This process, coupled with support, has been shown to reduce depressive symptoms.[36] An important feature of this approach is that it encourages patients to take a proactive position in their own care. In contrast, patients who cope by avoiding problems can have worsened depressive symptoms and often worse compliance. HF clinicians should familiarize themselves with available support groups in their area. Support group participation can be of value by providing additional education and by improving support. Mental health (MH) counseling has a role with these patients as well. There is evidence in the psychiatric literature that psychotherapy, especially cognitive behavioral therapy (CBT), can be of help in cases of mild to moderate depression. As such, clinicians should also consider referrals to MH providers. In cases of moderate to severe depression, HF providers should make a MH referral promptly and consider antidepressant medications. The Enhancing Recovery in Coronary Heart Disease (ENRICHD) study showed cognitive behavioral therapy reduced recurrent infarction and modestly reduced depression. However, it did not alter either general or cardiac mortality. In this regard, antidepressant medications can confer mortality benefits.[37,38]

There is ample evidence to show selective serotonin reuptake inhibitors (SSRIs) are safe and effective in cardiac patients with depressive symptoms. Clinicians should consider antidepressant medications as an important part of their cardiac treatment armamentarium. While the studies in cardiac patients have examined fluoxetine, paroxetine, sertraline, and others, three of the SSRIs – sertraline, escitalopram, and citalopram – are less likely to inhibit the cytochrome P450 system and hence other medication levels. Citalopram can inhibit beta-blocker metabolism so care should be taken when starting it in patients already on beta-blockers. HF clinicians can consider the use of these specific SSRIs when an antidepressant is indicated.

Anxiety comes in many forms, and can be a normative response to threatening situations. In this regard, some degree of anxiety in the presence of declines in health or escalating numbers of tests and procedures is normative. But some patients find themselves unable to cope with the burgeoning onslaught of health problems and life changes. Friedman found 36% of chronic heart failure outpatients had symptoms of anxiety.[31] When present, anxiety is known to increase the risk of CHD.[23]

Anxiety syndromes are also important to identify. These can include panic disorder, acute stress disorder (ASD), and posttraumatic stress disorder (PTSD). Panic disorder is characterized by recurring intense panic attacks that come on without warning. If precipitants are present, the panic symptoms are significantly out of proportion to the triggering event or circumstance. Physiological symptoms can include racing heart, a feeling of not being able to get enough air, lightheadedness, a choking sensation or lump in the throat, chest pains, and others. In addition, patients can believe they are going crazy or are about to die. The panic attacks usually pass in minutes, but can leave patients with lingering fear, often about the places the panic attacks occur. This lingering fear can restrict patients from going back to those places, or in severe cases even from venturing out of the house at all.

ASD and PTSD can develop in some patients who receive shocks from their intracardiac defibrillators. These two anxiety syndromes have similar symptom pictures. Symptoms can include flashbacks or dreams of the ICD shocks, marked avoidance of situations that could lead to a shock, or places where a shock occurred significant anxiety about possible future firings, disruption of daily tasks due to the anxiety, resultant sleep problems, irritability/outbursts, diminished concentration, and an increased startle response. However, they differ in their time courses. In ASD, symptoms begin within 1 month of the shocks and last for no more than a month, whereas PTSD symptoms begin within 3 months of a shock and can be ongoing. Additional diagnostic criteria for these and panic disorder can be found in the Diagnostic and Statistical Manual of Mental Disorders, Fourth Edition.[39]

Interventions for anxiety can include mental health referrals. Counseling can be of help as a means of support, by exploring underlying and contributing psychological factors, and by teaching coping strategies. In some cases, MH providers can teach specific relaxation techniques. HF clinicians would do well to familiarize themselves with MH providers in their area who have experience in treating anxiety symptoms.

Interventions for anxiety can also include medications. Benzodiazepines have a limited role because of their potential for sedation, which can cause further impairment in cognitive function as well as reduction in muscular coordination in already weakened patients. If used, lorazepam and oxazepam should be considered. These specific benzodiazepines undergo Phase 2 metabolism, so are not susceptible to enzymatic inhibition via the cytochrome P450 system, and have no active metabolites to accumulate. SSRIs are well known to have some anxiolytic effects, so these can also be considered when treating anxiety in this population. Clinicians should be aware that while antidepressant effects of the SSRIs can take four or more weeks to appear, the anxiolytic effects can be seen within a week or two.

References

1. Lown B, DeSilva RA, Reich P, et al. (1980) Psychophysiologic factors in sudden cardiac death. Am J Psychiatry 137:1325–1335
2. Chang PP, Ford DE, Meoni LA, et al. (2002) Anger in young men and subsequent premature cardiovascular disease: the precursors study. Arch Int Med 162:901–906
3. Eaker ED, Sullivan LM, Kelly-Hayes M, et al. (2004) Anger and hostility predict development of atrial fibrillation in men in the Framingham Offspring Study. Circulation 109:1267–1271
4. Kawachi I, Sparrow D, Spiro A, et al. (1996) A prospective study of anger and coronary artery disease. The Normative Aging Study. Circulation 94:2090–2095

5. Williams JE, Paton CC, Siegler IC, et al. (2000) Anger proneness predicts coronary heart disease risk: prospective analysis from the Atherosclerosis Risk in Communities (ARIC) Study. Circulation 101:2034–2039

6. Williams JE, Nieto FJ, Sanford CP, et al. (2001) Effects of an angry temperament on coronary heart disease risk: the Atherosclerosis Risk in Communities Study. Am J Epidemiol 154:230–235

7. Burg MM, Jain D, Soufer R, et al. (1993) Role of behavioral and psychological factors in mental stress-induced silent left ventricular dysfunction in coronary artery disease. Am J Coll Cardiol 22:440–448

8. Burg MM, Vashist A, Soufer R (2005) Mental stress ischemia: present status and future goals. J Nucl Cardiol 12:523–529

9. Sheps DS, McMahon RP, Becker L, et al. (2002) Mental stress-induced ischemia and all-cause mortality in patients with coronary artery disease: results from the Psychological Investigations of Myocardial Ischemia study. Circulation 105:1780–1784

10. Mittelman MA, Maclure M, Sherwood JB, et al. (1995) Triggering of acute myocardial infarction onset by episodes of anger. Determinants of Myocardial Infarction Onset Study Investigators. Circulation 92:1720–1725

11. Yusuf S, Hawken S, Ounpuu S, et al. (2004) Effect of potentially modifiable risk factors associated with myocardial infarction in 52 counties (the INTREHEART study): case-control study. Lancet 364:937–952

12. Case RB, Moss AJ, Case N, et al. (1992) Living alone after myocardial infarction: impact on prognosis. J Am Med Assoc 267:515–519

13. Krumholz HM, Butler J, Miller J (1998) Prognostic importance of emotional support for elderly patients hospitalized with heart failure. Circulation 97:958–964

14. Evangelista LS, Berg J, Dracup K (2001) Relationship between psychosocial variables and compliance in patients with heart failure. Heart Lung 30:294–301

15. Benson H, Alexander S, Feldman CL (1975) Decreased premature ventricular contractions through the use of relaxation response in patients with stable ischemic heart disease. Lancet 2:380–382

16. Langosch W, Seer P, Brodner G, et al. (1982) Behavior therapy with coronary heart disease patients: results of a comparative study. J Psychosom Res 26:475–484

17. Kubzansky LD, Sparrow D, Vokonas P, et al. (2001) Is the glass half empty of half full? A prospective study of optimism and coronary heart disease in the Normative Aging Study. Psychosom Med 63:910–916

18. Dickson VV, Tkacs N, Riegel B (2007) Cognitive influences on self-care decision making in person with heart failure. Am Heart J 154(3):424–431

19. Yalom ID (1985) The Theory and Practice of Group Psychotherapy. Basic Books, New York, NY

20. Gruen W (1975) Effects of psychotherapy during the hospitalization period on the recovery process in heart attacks. J Consult Clin Psychol 43:274–290

21. Oldenburg B, Perkins RJ, Andrews G (1985) Controlled trial of psychological intervention in myocardial infarction. J Consult Clin Psychol 53: 852–859

22. Luttik ML, Blaauwbroek A, Dijker A, et al. (2007) Living with heart failure: partner perspectives. J Cardiovasc Nurs 22(2):131–137

23. Kubzansky LD (2007) Sick at heart: the pathophysiology of negative emotions. Clev Clin J Med 74(suppl 1):S67–S72

24. Powell LH, Catellier D, Freedland KE, et al. (2005) Depression and heart failure in patients with a new myocardial infarction. Am Heart J 149(5):851–855

25. Sherwood A, Blumenthal JA, Trivedi R, et al. (2007) Relationship of depression to death or hospitalization in patients with heart failure. Arch Int Med 167:367–373

26. Abramson J, Berger A, Krumholz HM, et al. (2001) Depression and risk of heart failure among older persons with isolated systolic hypertension. Arch Int Med 161:1725–1730

27. Rumsfeld JS, Havranek E, Masoudi FA, et al. (2003) Depressive symptoms are the strongest predictors of short-term declines in health status in patients with heart failure. J Am Coll Cardiol 42:1811–1817

28. Joynt KE, Whellan DJ, O#x0027;Connor CM (2003) Depression and cardiovascular disease: mechanisms of interaction. Biol Psychiatry 54:248 261

29. Ziegelstein RC, Fauerbach JA, Stevens SS, et al. (2000) Patients with depression are less likely to follow recommendations to reduce cardiac risk during recovery from a myocardial infarction. Arch Int Med 160:1818–1823

30. Jiang W, Alexander J, Christopher E, et al. (2001) Relationship of depression to increased risk of mortality and rehospitalization in patients with congestive heart failure. Arch Int Med 161:1849–1856

31. Freidmann E, Thomas SA, Liu F, et al. (2006) Relationship of depression, anxiety, and social isolation to chronic heart failure outpatient mortality. Am Heart J 152:940.e1–e8

32. Kroenke K, Spitzer RL, Williams JB (2001) The PHQ-9: validity of a brief depression severity measure. J Gen Intern Med 16(9):606–613

33. Beck AT, Steer RA (1987) Beck Depression Inventory Manual. Psychological Corporation, San Antonio, TX

34. Hamilton M (1960) A rating scale for depression. J Neurol Neurosurg Psychiatry 23:56–62

35. Havranek EP, Spertus JA, Masoudi FA, et al. (2004) Predictors of the onset of depressive symptoms in patients with heart failure. J Am Coll Cardiol 44:2333–2338

36. Vollman MW, Lamontagne LL, Hepworth JT (2007) Coping and depressive symptoms in adults living with heart failure. J Cardiovasc Nurs 22(2):125–130

37. Glassman AH (2005) Does treating post-myocardial infarction depression reduce medical mortality? Arch Gen Psychiatry 62:711–712
38. Taylor CB, Youngblood ME, Catellier D, et al. (2005) Effects of antidepressant medication on morbidity and mortality in depressed patients after myocardial infarction. Arch Gen Psychiatry 62:792–798
39. American Psychiatric Association (1994) Diagnostic and Statistical Manual for Mental Disorders, Fourth Edition. American Psychiatric Association, Washington DC

Chapter 18
Inpatient Nursing Management

Heidi Kipp, Lisa Musshafen, and Lisa Norsen

INTRODUCTION

The role of the nurses and the multidisciplinary team in the successful management of inpatients being treated for heart failure (HF) should not be minimized. The attention of skilled and competent staff assures that HF patients progress according to an established plan of care, achieve optimal outcomes, and are fully prepared for discharge and smooth transition into the community. The purpose of this chapter is to outline important aspects of inpatient care and to detail the significant contributions of specialized nursing staff and a multidisciplinary heart failure and transplant team HFTT.

Optimally, inpatient care of individuals with heart failure is best managed by a heart failure and transplant team (HFTT). This multidisciplinary team works effectively to assure that patients receive optimal care and move efficiently though the system. Central to the success of the heart failure team is specially trained nursing staff and nurse practitioners. Their contributions to patient intake, daily management, and discharge ensure effective and timely care. In addition, the team works collaboratively to improve patient, provider, and system outcomes.

Statement of Need

Heart failure is a chronic disease affecting over five million people.[1,2] It accounts for over 990,000 inpatient admissions per year[3] and is the leading cause of hospital (re)admission in older adults.[4] Heart failure is a disabling condition that burdens not only the patient but their caregivers, and society. An estimated ten billion

J.D. Bisognano et al. (eds.), *Manual of Heart Failure Management,*
DOI: 10.1007/978-1-84882-185-9_18, © Springer-Verlag London Limited 2009

dollars is spent annually to diagnose, treat, and manage HF and experts predict that this amount will increase as treatment options expand and patients live longer with the disease.[4,5] Hospitalizations account for over 75% of the cost of care and highlight the imperative that inpatient management be efficient and effective.

INPATIENT CARE

Admission

Many patients with HF are managed successfully for many years by primary care physicians in the community. Referral to a cardiologist should occur whenever treatment of initial symptoms is refractory to standard therapies such as vasodilators, diuretics, ACE inhibitors, and/or digoxin.[3] There is growing evidence that early referral to outpatient case management programs (specialized heart failure and transplant services) is beneficial for the patient in terms of symptom management and longevity, and the system in terms of reducing hospital readmissions and cost.[6]

Indications for hospitalization are outlined elsewhere.[7] Access to specialized inpatient care occurs through various portals of entry including referral from physician offices, outpatient specialty clinics, regional or community hospitals, and emergency departments (ED). When possible, bypassing ED through direct referral to the HFTT should be encouraged. Direct referral is facilitated by developing broad-based community knowledge about referral criteria and the availability and benefits of specialty services, and assuring "user friendly" systems to connect community providers, clinics, and hospitals to heart failure/transplant specialists.

When a patient is seen in the ED, the first priority is to determine level of care: intensive care, specialty care, or general care.[8] Admission to the heart failure service should be considered if the patient has had several inpatient admissions for HF management, has failed to improve clinically despite treatment, has HF with left ventricular dysfunction, a new murmur, abnormal renal function, uncontrolled hypertension, ongoing ischemia, or HF with shock.[8] Once accepted by the HF service, prompt admission to the HF unit is essential.

Intake

Once the patient has been admitted to the heart failure and transplant unit, specially trained nursing staff begin their evaluation of physiological and psychosocial needs. Standardized tools, such as intake forms (Figure 18.1) and advance directives (Figure 18.2), assist the nurse in collecting consistent data that details important information needed to formulate the inpatient plan of care and to commence discharge teaching. The patient's family and/or support network is included from the outset since patient and family education is the foundation of successful long-term HF management. For example, patients are instructed about daily weights and strict

a

STRONG HEALTH
STRONG MEMORIAL HOSPITAL

ADULT INTERDISCIPLINARY RISK SCREEN
SMH 423 MR Page 1 of 2
CONTINUITY OF CARE
RN to complete all assessments (shaded areas) on form

☐ Inpatient
☐ Outpatient
☐ Strong Surgical Center

The following forms, if available, must be reviewed prior to completion of this Screen: Ambulatory Medicine Adult Interdisciplinary Health Assessment/Risk Screen; ED Transfer Form; Preadmission Continuity of Care (PACCT) Form; History and Physical; Medication List; and Face Sheet.

SECTION I:

Admitting Unit: ____ Today's Date: ____ Time: ____ am/pm Source of Data: ____

☐ **Patient rights reviewed with / patient / patient representative.** ☐ **Given Admission Information Packet.**

ADVANCE DIRECTIVES (AD) SCREEN:
☐ Yes ☐ No Has an Advance Directive(s)?
If yes, type: ☐ Health Care Proxy ☐ Living Will ☐ DNR ☐ Other: ____
If yes, Advance Directive available for inclusion in the chart? ☐ Yes ☐ No (If not, new Advance Directive to be completed)
☐ Yes ☐ No Would like to complete a Health Care Proxy form?
☐ Yes ☐ No Would like information about Advance Directives? If yes, given: ☐ Health Care Proxy ☐ AD Information
Assessment: ☐ AD placed in chart ☐ Consult with appropriate medical provider for completion of new AD
☐ AD teaching done ☐ No action needed (Has answered "no" to all questions)

CONTAGION SCREEN:
☐ Need for contagion precautions (specify): ____
☐ Influenza vaccine this fall/winter: ☐ Yes ☐ No ☐ Unknown ☐ N/A
☐ Pneumonia vaccine: ☐ Yes ☐ No ☐ Unknown
Assessment: ☐ Isolation required ☐ HO/NP notified ☐ No need identified

SMOKING CESSATION SCREEN:
☐ Yes ☐ No Has smoked within the last year?
Assessment: ☐ If Yes: ☐ Advised that SMH is a smoke-free environment ☐ Counseled to stop smoking ☐ Given printed smoking cessation information
☐ If No, no action needed

LATEX SCREEN:
☐ Yes ☐ No Allergy to latex or rubber products
☐ Yes ☐ No Reaction such as hives, swelling or difficulty breathing after contact with rubber products
☐ Yes ☐ No Currently on latex precautions
If "Yes" to any of the above questions, notify the MD/NP and institute latex precautions until/unless MD/NP gives specific order.
Assessment: ☐ Notify MD/NP and place on latex precautions ☐ No need identified

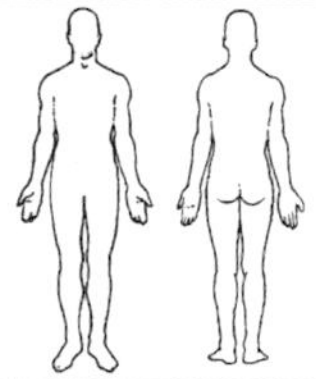

VISUAL SKIN SCREEN:
Document the number of any skin breakdown or injury* on the diagram:
1. Wound/Ulcer 2. Rash 3. Reddened area
4. Laceration 5. Burn 6. Ecchymosis
7. Bite 8. Old injury 9. Other: ____
*Note required for any identified skin breakdown / injury
Assessment: ☐ No skin breakdown / injury noted ☐ Note written

PAIN / FUNCTIONAL SCREEN:
☐ Yes ☐ No Pain in the past 24 hours? Location: ☐ Head ☐ Neck or shoulders ☐ Upper extremities ☐ Chest ☐ Upper back ☐ Abdomen or pelvis ☐ Low back or buttocks ☐ Lower extremities
Using pain scale, how much pain now? ____ How long have you had pain? ____ What helps relieve the pain? ____
Using pain scale, worst level of pain within the past seven days? ____ Your goal for pain relief (0-10 scale): ____
☐ Yes ☐ No Would you like us to develop a pain treatment plan for you? ____
☐ Yes ☐ No Identified weakness/paralysis/neuropathy If yes, specify if cause known: ____
Activities that you can do independently: ☐ Getting out of a chair ☐ Walking ☐ Dressing ☐ Cooking ☐ Climbing stairs ☐ Bathing ☐ Toileting ☐ Feeding yourself ☐ Work or other daily activities
☐ Yes ☐ No Does pain interfere with your ability to do daily activities?
Housing: ☐ No home ☐ Apartment ☐ House ☐ One-level ☐ Multi-level ☐ Other ____
Adaptive equipment (document on SMH 43 MR if equipment with patient): ☐ Glasses ☐ Hearing Aid ☐ Cane ☐ Walker ☐ Prosthesis ☐ Splint ☐ Other ____
Who lives with you? ____ Location of bedroom: ____ Location of bathroom: ____
Assessment:
If any risk factor is identified, refer to MD/NP for pain treatment plan or to consider PT/OT consult.
☐ Referral made to: ____ Date/Time: ____ Signature: ____ ☐ No need identified

Signature / Title of RN / LPN / PA Obtaining Section 1 Data: ____	*Date/ Time:* ____	*Signature / Title of RN / LPN / PA Updating Section 1 Data:* ____	*Date/ Time:* ____
Signature / Title of RN / PA Completing Section 1 Assessment: ____	*Date/ Time:* ____	*Signature / Title of RN / PA Updating Section 1 Assessment:* ____	*Date/ Time:* ____

Rev. 8/06

FIGURE 18.1. (**a**) Nursing adult interdisciplinary risk screen page 1. (**b**) Nursing adult interdisciplinary risk screen page 2.

b Patient Name: _____   **SMH 423 MR**   Page 2 of 2

SECTION II:

Height: _____ Weight: _____ **kg** Scale Type: _____

ALLERGIES: ☐ *If yes, Red Alert Band on patient and allergies clearly stated*
Medication Allergies to prescriptions, over-the-counter drugs, vitamins, herbal supplements:

☐ Yes* ☐ No   If 'Yes', specify _____

Other Adverse Effects: ☐ Yes* ☐ No   If 'Yes', specify _____

Other Allergies: ☐ Yes* ☐ No   If 'Yes', specify _____

Assessment: ☐ Reviewed by RN

MODIFIED BRADEN SCALE:

RISK ASSESSMENT	1	2	3	4	SCORE
SENSORY PERCEPTION	1 Unresponsive to painful stimuli	2 Responds only to painful stimuli, sensory impairment over 1/2 Body	3 Can't communicate need to turn or sensory impairment in 1 or 2 extremities	4 No sensory impairment	
MOISTURE	1 Constantly moist by perspiration, urine	2 Moist, change linens 1x Per Shift	3 Occasionally moist, extra linen change once a day	4 Rarely moist, routine linen change	
ACTIVITY	1 Bedfast	2 Chairfast	3 Walks occasionally	4 Walks frequently	
MOBILITY	1 Completely immobile	2 Very limited, occasional slight change in position	3 Slightly limited, frequent but slight position change	4 No Major Limitations, Frequent Position Change	
NUTRITION	1 Very poor, Never Eats Complete Meal	2 Probably inadequate, eats About 1/2 food	3 Adequate eats over 1/2 Food	4 Excellent, eats most of food	
FRICTION & SHEAR	1 Moderate to Maximum assistance in Moving	2 Requires minimal assistance to move	3 Moves independently	4	

TOTAL SCORE

Assessment: Total Score < 16: Implement SMH 1362A Nursing Protocol: Potential Alteration in Skin Integrity
Pressure Sore Present: Implement SMH 1382B Nursing Protocol: Actual Alteration in Skin Integrity
If patient has a Stage III or Stage IV ulcer present, ask HO to consider a consult by a physician in Plastic Surgery.

☐ Referral made to: _____ Date/Time: _____ Signature: _____
☐ No need identified

NUTRITION / METABOLISM SCREEN:

Usual Diet: _____ ☐ Appetite: _____ ☐ Religious, cultural or personal food preferences _____
☐ Unintentional weight loss or gain of > 4.5 kg or 5% of body weight in past month   ☐ Tube feedings
☐ Aspiration or significant problems chewing / swallowing   ☐ New occurrence of draining wound/fistula/skin breakdown/decubitus
☐ Nausea / vomiting / diarrhea / constipation > 2 weeks   ☐ Pregnant or lactating woman admitted for a medical problem
☐ Severe food allergy / intolerance (list) _____
☐ Patient and/or Significant Other have not previously received education on special diet prior to admission.

Assessment:
If a risk factor is identified, refer: a) nutritional risk factor to Registered Dietitian at x7-1700 and   b) speech/swallowing factor to MD/NP to consider Speech Consult.
☐ Referral made to: _____ Date/Time: _____ Signature: _____
☐ No need identified

SPIRITUAL / CULTURAL NEEDS:
☐ Requests visit from clergy ☐ Any treatments or situations that your beliefs would prohibit? _____ ☐ Special Needs: _____
Assessment: ☐ Referral made at x5-2187 to: _____ Date/Time: _____ Signature: _____ ☐ None

INITIAL DISCHARGE PLAN / PSYCHOSOCIAL RISK SCREEN:

☐ Yes ☐ No   CARE GIVER ISSUES: (e.g., Absence of social supports; Guardian unable to give adequate care; Cognitive impairment; Involvement with the law; Personal or family crisis in progress including recent traumatic loss, personal instability, family conflict)

☐ Yes ☐ No   USE OF HEALTH CARE SERVICES: (e.g., Non-compliance with medications, appointments, diet or other health care recommendations; Frequent ED visits, hospital admissions within past six months; Prior or current utilization of home health care services; Readmission within 72 hours of discharge)

☐ Yes ☐ No   HIGH RISK ISSUES: (e.g., Domestic violence; Suspected abuse/neglect; Patient abduction; Life threatening illness/injury; Substance abuse (patient/family); Suicide / homicide potential (patient/family)

☐ Yes ☐ No   RESOURCE NEEDS: (e.g., Lack of concrete resources (housing, food, clothing, insurance); Homeless (no known address, phone number); Language or other cultural barriers; Frail or homebound, living alone; Unable to provide or plan for adequate self-care, e.g., ADL's)

☐ Yes ☐ No   DISPOSITION: (e.g., Admitted from long term care / institutional setting; Possible discharge to alternate setting, including rehab, nursing facility)

If 'Yes' to any factor briefly specify details: _____

Assessment: If a risk factor is identified, referral to Social Worker is required. Notification Protocol: Days Monday-Friday notify unit Social Worker immediately via pager; Evenings via phone/mail; and weekends via page office for covering social worker.
☐ Referral made to: _____ Date/Time: _____ Signature: _____
☐ No need identified

Signature / Title of RN / LPN / PA	Date/	Signature / Title of RN / LPN / PA	Date/
Obtaining Data:	Time:	Updating Data:	Time:
Signature / Title of RN / PA	Date/	Signature / Title of RN / PA	Date/
Completing Assessment:	Time:	Updating Assessment:	Time:

KEY: PA - Physician Assistant

FIGURE 18.1. (continued)

intake and output (I & O) records. If patients are able, they take
responsibility for keeping track of their I & O and the nurse checks
the records every 4–8 h. When checking weights and I & O, the
nurse discusses management of weight gain and deviations in
I & O. Self care is stressed through out hospitalization so that the
transition to home care is seamless.

STRONG 🝔 HEALTH
STRONG MEMORIAL HOSPITAL

CONTINUITY OF CARE
SMH **1094 MR**

**Advanced Directives
Tracking Form**

☐ Inpatient   ☐ Outpatient

1. Has the Patient completed an Advance Directive document(s)?
   A. Health Care Proxy   ☐ Yes, Date signed: _____ ☐ No
   B. Living Will   ☐ Yes, Date signed: _____ ☐ No
   C. DNR   ☐ Yes, Date signed: _____ ☐ No
   D. Other: _____

2. If the patient has an Advance Directive(s), is there a copy in the patient's current inpatient medical chart?
   ☐ Yes   ☐ No
   If no, who will obtain document? (specify) _____ Date Expected: _____ Date Received:_____

3. If the patient does not have an Advance Directive, has the patient/family member received Health Care
   Proxy/Advance Directive(s) information?
   ☐ Yes   ☐ No
   If yes, provided by whom:_____ Date: _____
   If no, please explain: _____
   _____
   _____
   _____
   _____
   _____

4. Who is the appointed agent (proxy) for health care decisions including DNR?

   Name:_____ Telephone: _____ Relationship to Patient: _____

5. Patient/family member requests additional information from a health care professional. ☐ Yes   ☐ No
   Name and date health care professional called:

   ☐ Physician   _____   _____
   ☐ Resident   _____   _____
   ☐ Nurse Practitioner   _____   _____
   ☐ Registered Nurse   _____   _____
   ☐ Social Worker   _____   _____
   ☐ Ethics Consultant (5-5800) _____   _____

   _____   _____
   RN Initiating form   Date

Rev. 7/98

FIGURE 18.2. Advanced directive tracking form.

All patients are seen by a heart failure nurse practitioner (NP) or a heart failure fellow. A complete history and physical is performed with a more detailed focus on heart failure symptoms and risk factors. Heart failure standard admission order sets are useful tools to assure consistent care and, ideally, are available in a clinical information system. An example of a standard order set is contained in Figure 18.3. The NPs review all home medications with the patient and/or family. Medication reconciliation is completed on admission and again upon transfers of care and at discharge. Ideally, reconciliation is done electronically so that changes and adjustments are available to all providers in real time and can be tracked across time.

The NP and/or fellow reviews the patient's information with the heart failure attending cardiologist and a plan of care is developed. The plan of care is individualized according to the patient's presentation and may be as simple as diuresis and uptitration of medications or include a battery of tests and surgical evaluation to determine treatment options. The attending physician, the NP, and the nurse take joint responsibility for communicating the plan of care to the patient and family (within the guidelines of HIPPA). Precise communication within this group is crucial so that patients receive a coherent and uniform message. Writing out the daily plan of care is desirable and can be accomplished easily by using dry erase boards at the bedside. If testing off the unit is indicated, portable monitoring may be necessary because of the increased risk of arrhythmias in this population. If portable monitoring is necessary, the patient should be accompanied by a nurse or other provider. The daily staffing plan should be created with this in mind.

Ongoing Management

The patient's plan of care and goals for discharge are re-evaluated daily at multidisciplinary care rounds or the "huddle." These occur 7 days a week and are facilitated by the attending cardiologist. All members of the HFTT are expected to attend. First on the agenda is a review of the patient's progress and discussion of pertinent issues or changes in patient's condition occurring over the previous 24 h. Next, both long- and short-term goals are reviewed, evaluated and modified to promote patient progress along the plan of care and to facilitate timely and safe discharge. Daily goal sheets help to keep the focus of care organized and provide reference for extended hospital stays (Figure 18.4). The discharge date is identified, reiterated, or modified daily during rounds so that all team members are working toward a common goal. The care coordinator (see discussion on multidisciplinary team in section "The Heart Failure Unit and Team") is responsible for summarizing the results of the huddle and enters the information discussed into an electronic document. The computerized document can be accessed and updated by all members of the team through-out the day.

a

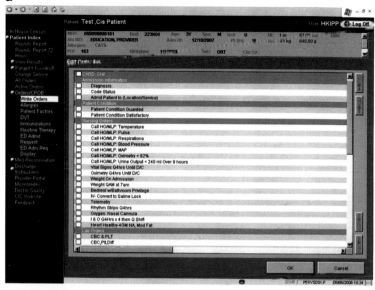

b

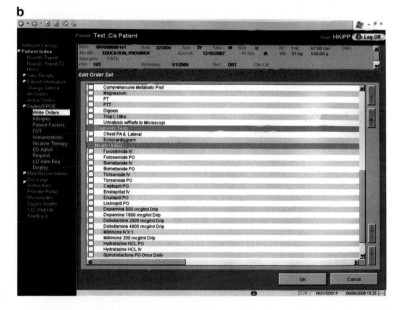

FIGURE 18.3. (a) Standardized heart failure orderset page 1. (b) Standardized heart failure orderset page 2.

a

STRONG ✸ HEALTH
STRONG MEMORIAL HOSPITAL

☒ Inpatient

ADULT CRITICAL CARE PATIENT GOAL SHEET/CARE PLAN AND PATIENT/FAMILY TEACHING RECORD

SMH 1361ICU MR

Page 1 of 2   Rev. 3/07

Admission Date: _____   Sheet # _____ of _____
Diagnosis: _____
Allergies: _____
Precautions: _____

➤ Goal Sheet/Care Plan sheet must be initiated upon admission to the ICU.
➤ For each identified health care need, circle the appropriate response (Y, N, N/A) to indicate whether intervention has been implemented or goal has been met. If goal is not met, document reason on flow sheet or in progress note.
➤ If intervention/goal marked with * does not apply to patient, charting does not need to be done in this area. Highlight area in yellow.
➤ Communicate any identified needs to the Health Care team during daily rounds. The Health Team includes: Physicians, Nurse Practitioners, Physician Assistants, Nurses, Respiratory Therapists, Nutritionists, Pharmacists, Social Workers, PT/OT, and Chaplains.
➤ Each shift must review the identified health care needs, interventions, goals, and sign.

Charting Codes
Y = Outcome met with or without nursing interventions. Reassess outcome every shift and prn.
    No additional documentation is needed.
N = This outcome is not met. Intervention required and supported with documentation in progress note, on Critical Care Flowsheet or on Medication Administration Record.
N/A= Does not apply

HEALTH CARE NEEDS	INTERVENTIONS/GOALS *Collaborate with health care team to revise interventions.	Date / Time	Date / Time	Date / Time	Date / Time	Date / Time	Date / Time	Date / Time
Medication Reconciliation	Have current medications been reviewed with team?	Y N	Y N	Y N	Y N	Y N	Y N	Y N
	Have home medications been reviewed with team?	Y N	Y N	Y N	Y N	Y N	Y N	Y N
Psychosocial/ Family	Family Update with team	Y N N/A	Y N N/A	Y N N/A	Y N N/A	Y N N/A	Y N N/A	Y N N/A
	Copy of Advance Directive in chart. Type _____	Y N	Y N	Y N	Y N	Y N	Y N	Y N
	Spiritual resources utilized	Y N N/A	Y N N/A	Y N N/A	Y N N/A	Y N N/A	Y N N/A	Y N N/A
	Referral/continued follow-up with social work if indicated	Y N N/A	Y N N/A	Y N N/A	Y N N/A	Y N N/A	Y N N/A	Y N N/A
Cardiovascular	Hemodynamics within prescribed limits	Y N	Y N	Y N	Y N	Y N	Y N	Y N
	Vasoactive agents at minimal effective dose for ordered parameters	Y N N/A	Y N N/A	Y N N/A	Y N N/A	Y N N/A	Y N N/A	Y N N/A
	*Aspirin, Statin, beta-Blocker, ACE-Inhibitor (circle)	Y N N/A	Y N N/A	Y N N/A	Y N N/A	Y N N/A	Y N N/A	Y N N/A
Respiratory (VAP Bundle)	HOB @ 30 degrees	Y N	Y N	Y N	Y N	Y N	Y N	Y N
	DVT Prophylaxis	Y N	Y N	Y N	Y N	Y N	Y N	Y N
	Peptic Ulcer Disease Prophylaxis	Y N	Y N	Y N	Y N	Y N	Y N	Y N
	Test for weaning or ability to extubate daily	Y N N/A	Y N N/A	Y N N/A	Y N N/A	Y N N/A	Y N N/A	Y N N/A
	Oral Care q 2 hours	Y N	Y N	Y N	Y N	Y N	Y N	Y N
	PT/OT initiated	Y N	Y N	Y N	Y N	Y N	Y N	Y N
	Mobility: at max activity level as tolerated	Y N	Y N	Y N	Y N	Y N	Y N	Y N
	Date Intubated _____ Extubated _____							
	*Evaluate for Trach Trach date _____	Y N N/A	Y N N/A	Y N N/A	Y N N/A	Y N N/A	Y N N/A	Y N N/A
Comfort: Pain/Sedation (VAP Bundle)	Sedation Scale: SAS 3-4	Y N	Y N	Y N	Y N	Y N	Y N	Y N
	Verbal Pain Scale < 4 or NVPS 0-2	Y N	Y N	Y N	Y N	Y N	Y N	Y N
	Sedation interrupted	Y N N/A	Y N N/A	Y N N/A	Y N N/A	Y N N/A	Y N N/A	Y N N/A
	Pain/Sedation medication weaning or at minimal dose	Y N	Y N	Y N	Y N	Y N	Y N	Y N
Neurological	*ICP within prescribed limits	Y N N/A	Y N N/A	Y N N/A	Y N N/A	Y N N/A	Y N N/A	Y N N/A
	*C-Spine Clearance	Y N N/A	Y N N/A	Y N N/A	Y N N/A	Y N N/A	Y N N/A	Y N N/A
Gastrointestinal	HAL / T-feed / Diet / NPO (circle)	Y N	Y N	Y N	Y N	Y N	Y N	Y N
	Nutrition at goal	Y N N/A	Y N N/A	Y N N/A	Y N N/A	Y N N/A	Y N N/A	Y N N/A
	Bowel Regimen ordered	Y N	Y N	Y N	Y N	Y N	Y N	Y N
	Last BM within 48 hours	Y N	Y N	Y N	Y N	Y N	Y N	Y N
Skin (Pressure Ulcer Bundle)	Without Pressure Ulcer	Y N	Y N	Y N	Y N	Y N	Y N	Y N
	If pressure ulcer present, documented on ICU Pressure Ulcer Flowsheet.	Y N N/A	Y N N/A	Y N N/A	Y N N/A	Y N N/A	Y N N/A	Y N N/A
	Braden Scale on Admission and Twice q week	SCORE:			SCORE:			
	Specialty bed / mattress type _____	Y N	Y N	Y N	Y N	Y N	Y N	Y N
Genitourinary (UTI Bundle)	Foley still required	Y N	Y N	Y N	Y N	Y N	Y N	Y N
	Output > Input	Y N	Y N	Y N	Y N	Y N	Y N	Y N
	*If No to above, Diuresis plan discussed?	Y N N/A	Y N N/A	Y N N/A	Y N N/A	Y N N/A	Y N N/A	Y N N/A
Endocrine	Insulin drip Protocol	Y N N/A	Y N N/A	Y N N/A	Y N N/A	Y N N/A	Y N N/A	Y N N/A
	Blood Glucose within target range ordered	Y N	Y N	Y N	Y N	Y N	Y N	Y N
Labs/ID (Central Line Bundle)	*Anemia Protocol	Y N N/A	Y N N/A	Y N N/A	Y N N/A	Y N N/A	Y N N/A	Y N N/A
	Frequency of lab draws addressed	Y N	Y N	Y N	Y N	Y N	Y N	Y N
	*Blood Saving Device utilized	Y N N/A	Y N N/A	Y N N/A	Y N N/A	Y N N/A	Y N N/A	Y N N/A
	Central line still required?	Y N N/A	Y N N/A	Y N N/A	Y N N/A	Y N N/A	Y N N/A	Y N N/A
Safety	ID/Allergy Band intact	Y N	Y N	Y N	Y N	Y N	Y N	Y N
	Restraint order current	Y N N/A	Y N N/A	Y N N/A	Y N N/A	Y N N/A	Y N N/A	Y N N/A
Other								
	Shift/Initials							
	Shift/Initials							
	Shift/Initials							

FIGURE 18.4. (**a**) Patient daily goal sheet and teaching record page 1. (**b**) Patient daily goal sheet and teaching record page 2.

b

STRONG 🎯 HEALTH
STRONG MEMORIAL HOSPITAL

**ADULT CRITICAL CARE PATIENT GOAL SHEET/CARE PLAN AND
PATIENT/FAMILY TEACHING RECORD**

SMH 1361ICU MR
Page 2 of 2

INTERDISCIPLINARY PLAN/SUMMARY OF GOALS

Date: _____	Date: _____	Date: _____	Date: _____
Provider Signature: _____	Provider Signature: _____	Provider Signature: _____	Provider Signature: _____
Date: _____	Date: _____	Date: _____	Date: _____
Provider Signature: _____	Provider Signature: _____	Provider Signature: _____	Provider Signature: _____

PATIENT/FAMILY EDUCATION PLAN AND TEACHING RECORD (RN initiates plan and RN/LPN provides teaching)

FACTORS/BARRIERS THAT AFFECT LEARNING: PATIENT ☐ No Barriers	FACTORS/BARRIERS THAT AFFECT LEARNING: FAMILY/SIGNIFICANT OTHER ☐ No Barriers
Physical: **Behavioral:** **Miscellaneous:** ☐ Vision Impairment ☐ Anxious ☐ Language ____ ☐ Hearing Impairment ☐ Intubated/Trach ☐ Cultural ____ ☐ Pain/Discomfort ☐ Uncooperative ☐ Age/Developmental ____ ☐ Learning Disability ☐ Severity of Illness ☐ Cognitive Impairments ☐ Other: ____	**Physical:** **Behavioral:** **Miscellaneous:** ☐ Vision Impairment ☐ Anxious ☐ Language ____ ☐ Hearing Impairment ☐ Withdrawn ☐ Literacy/Reading Skill ____ ☐ Speech Impairment ☐ Uncooperative ☐ Cultural/Religious ____ ☐ Learning Disability ☐ Other:

1. Person Taught Pt= Patient F = Family O = Other: ____	2. Current Understanding A = Verbalizes Accurately B = Needs Reinforcement C = None D = Expresses Understanding (nonverbal)	3. Readiness to Learn A = Asks Questions appropriately B = Anxious C = Uncooperative	4. Method D = Demonstration I = Individual Instruction T = Teaching sheet/pamphlet given (reviewed)	5. Outcome V = Verbalizes Accurately D = Demonstrates NR= Needs Reinforcement NV= Expresses Understanding (nonverbal)

Teaching Outcomes	1. Person Taught	2. Current Understanding	3. Readiness to Learn	4. Method	5. Outcome	Date & Initials	Reinforce Date & Initials	Reinforce Date & Initials	Reinforce Date & Initials	Reinforce Date & Initials	Reinforce Date & Initials	Reinforce Date & Initials	Comment
Plan for Care and Services:													
• Oriented to the ICU environment & visitor policy													
• Completes family spokesperson agreement													
• Explains reason for admission													
• Explains ICU physician coverage and consulting services													
• Describes members of the multidisciplinary team and their responsibilities: RT, PT, OT, SW, Nutrition, MD, RN, NP													
Treatment/Procedures													
• Explains patient's physical condition, monitoring and and use of supportive equipment													
• Describes tests and procedures													
Diet/Nutrition													
• Describes nutrition interventions; HAL/Enteral feedings													
Safety/Preventing Complications													
Discusses the following with patient/family/other													
• Mechanical ventilation: modes, weaning, tracheostomy													
• Mobility: dangle, OOB to chair													
• Skin: positioning, wound care, specialty mattress													
• Medications: names, actions, side effects													
Pain/Other Symptom Management													
• Describes pain, symptom assessment system													
• Explains medications to relieve pain/other symptoms													
Review "Smoke Free Inside and Out" with patient/family/other													
Other													
Cardiac Surgery teaching booklet Sternal precautions reviewed													

Initials	Full Signature	Title	Initials	Full Signature	Title	Initials	Full Signature	Title

KEY: HAL - Hyperalimentation   NVPS - Nonverbal Pain Scale   SAS - Sedation Agitation Scale

FIGURE 18.4. (continued)

Facilitating goal directed care is an important, albeit complicated, undertaking and the unit-based NP is central to its success. Essential daily tasks include reviewing and updating medications and standing orders such as lab work, advancing patient care such as diet and activity, follow up on all ordered tests and procedures, prioritizing, and queuing new tests, procedures, and treatments, and assuring patient comfort and safety such as initiating appropriate protocols for prevention of skin breakdown and prevention of falls.

Discharge Planning and Patient Education

Discharge planning is started at the time of admission and must be addressed daily. Discharge barriers are discussed during rounds and team members are assigned responsibility to resolve specific issues and report back to the team. Care must be taken to ensure that a safe discharge plan is in place and that appropriate options are available to meet the needs of the patient: home plan with or without community referrals, short-term rehabilitation, long-term placement, or palliative or hospice care. If the discharge plan is complex, the multidisciplinary team should schedule a family meeting to clarify goals of care, to define the plan of care, and to formulate a safe and realistic discharge plan. At all junctures, patients and families should be involved in the discharge planning process.

Patient education is the centerpiece of inpatient care and outpatient management of HF. Nurses and NPs play a pivotal role in orchestrating patient education and assessing achievement of desired outcomes. A comprehensive, individualized education plan must be in place for all HF patients. Documentation of progress toward educational goals should be accessible to all team members. Patients receive multiple educational tools as part of the discharge process but the standardized teaching tool for HF patients is the Symptom Awareness Tool with a weight monitoring grid (Figure 18.5). In addition to the Symptom Awareness Tool, the patient receives a copy of their personalized discharge instructions related to activity, diet, medication regimen, and follow up appointments.

CONSULTS AND REFERRALS

The HFTT must maintain close working relationships with multiple consult services. While the decision to consult is usually made by the multidisciplinary team or attending physician, it is often the responsibility of the NP to initiate and follow up on consults. The electrophysiology, nephrology, endocrine, and palliative care services are most often consulted because of the disease trajectory and comor-

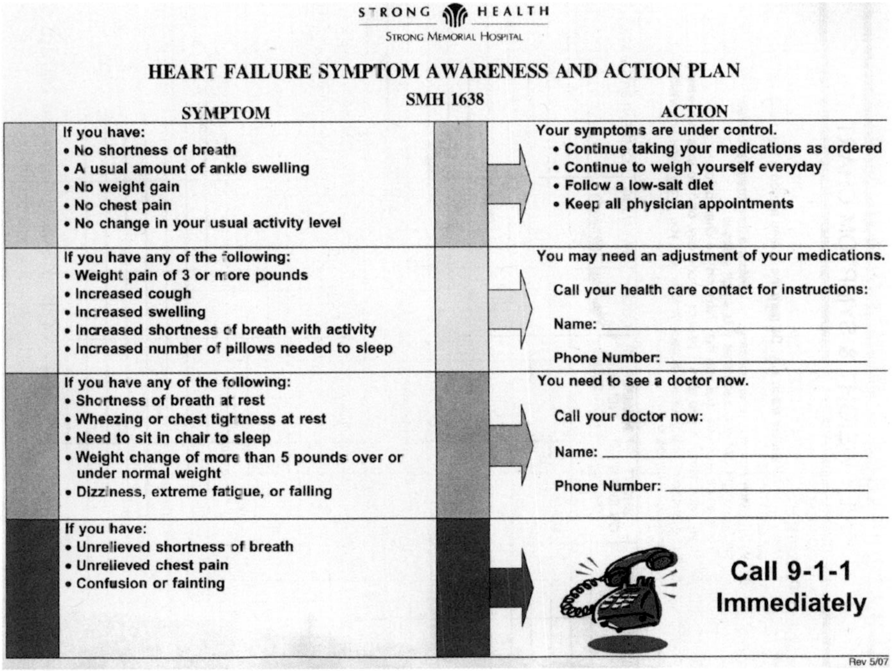

STRONG ✺ HEALTH
STRONG MEMORIAL HOSPITAL

HEART FAILURE SYMPTOM AWARENESS AND ACTION PLAN

SMH 1638

SYMPTOM	ACTION

If you have:
- No shortness of breath
- A usual amount of ankle swelling
- No weight gain
- No chest pain
- No change in your usual activity level

→ **Your symptoms are under control.**
- Continue taking your medications as ordered
- Continue to weigh yourself everyday
- Follow a low-salt diet
- Keep all physician appointments

If you have any of the following:
- Weight pain of 3 or more pounds
- Increased cough
- Increased swelling
- Increased shortness of breath with activity
- Increased number of pillows needed to sleep

→ **You may need an adjustment of your medications.**
Call your health care contact for instructions:
Name: _____
Phone Number: _____

If you have any of the following:
- Shortness of breath at rest
- Wheezing or chest tightness at rest
- Need to sit in chair to sleep
- Weight change of more than 5 pounds over or under normal weight
- Dizziness, extreme fatigue, or fainting

→ **You need to see a doctor now.**
Call your doctor now:
Name: _____
Phone Number: _____

If you have:
- Unrelieved shortness of breath
- Unrelieved chest pain
- Confusion or fainting

→ **Call 9-1-1
Immediately**

Rev 5/07

FIGURE 18.5. (a) Patient education tool: Heart failure symptom awareness and action plan. (b) Patient education tool: Daily weight and symptom chart.

b

DAILY WEIGHT & SYMPTOM CHART

Instructions:
1. Use the same scales each day. Be sure the scales are on a flat, hard surface.
2. Weigh each morning after urinating, but before eating breakfast. Wear similar weight clothing each time you weigh yourself.
3. Check any symptoms that you may have on the chart below.
4. Notify your doctor if you gain 3 pounds in one day, or 5 pounds in a week.
5. Bring this form and your medication bottles with you _every_ time you visit the clinic or hospital!

DATE	WEIGHT	SHORT OR BREATH (Yes/No)	NUMBER OF PILLOWS FOR SLEEP	COUGH (Yes/No)	SWELLING (Where?)	COMMENTS/QUESTIONS

FIGURE 18.5. (continued).

bidities associated with HF. Formal referral is preferred for complex and ongoing issues, but "curbside" consulting is a valuable tool in facilitating care. Building and maintaining strong relationships with consulting services is indispensable in day-to-day management.

Subspecialty teams often have NPs or educators who can commit time and resource to meeting the needs of the HF patients. For example, the endocrine service may have an educator who can direct the unit staff in planning for timely discharge of the newly diagnosed diabetic.

INVASIVE MONITORING

Heart failure patients may require continuous hemodynamic monitoring with Swan-Ganz catheters. Such monitoring is no longer an indication for ICU level care but does require special training and enhanced staffing levels called step down or intermediate level care. The advantages of invasive monitoring on a step down unit are many. Patients are typically more mobile and can retain a near normal pattern of activity and visitation. Maintaining invasive monitoring on the unit means less disruption in care for patients and families. As is often the case, HF patients establish important relationships with unit staff and continuity of their provider team is maintained. Special considerations for patients with Swan-Ganz catheters include confirming placement by checking and recording depths at least every 8 h and before and after each ambulation or movement from bed to chair, evaluating waveforms every 2 h, and checking an X-ray after placement and then twice weekly, and with any change in swan depth.

DEVICE MANAGEMENT

After evaluating the patient's response to treatments, it may be necessary to pursue surgical options. If surgical options are necessary and appropriate for the patient, the specialized HF floor can accommodate the needs of these patients without disrupting the care team or the care plan. Nursing staff is educated and trained to take care of surgical patients before and after surgery (except for ICU level care). The patients can include post high-risk coronary artery bypass grafting with persistent decreased left ventricular function, post heart transplant, and post ventricular assist devices (VAD). The nurses undergo initial VAD and heart transplant training once they have demonstrated competence in caring for HF patients, usually about 6 months after initial hire. After initial training, yearly competencies are maintained. Nurse practitioners need extensive training in VAD management and should be fully facile in handling VAD emergencies. This highly specialized area of care requires cooperation with the VAD coordinators who are trained and dedicated to the care of VAD patients.

NURSING STAFFING

The HF unit is staffed by specially trained, expert nursing staff. Their expertise assures the delivery of safe, high-quality care. The work of providing nursing care is defined in different ways including nursing care hours per patient day (NCHPPD), patient to nurse staffing ratios, and variable staffing based on acuity indices. Each methodology acknowledges that different patients have different nursing needs and that the staffing models must reflect this need. NCHPPD is a widely accepted methodology and provides some flexibility in meeting daily staffing needs. When using the NCHPPD methodology it is important to account for the types of patients (Swan-Ganz, device, vasoactive drips, etc.) *and* the daily census of each type of patient served on the unit. The sickest patients (i.e., Swan-Ganz and device) require a NCHPPD designation of 18–20 NCHPPD; those patients on vasoactive drips are designated at 8–12 NCHPPD; and general care patients require 6–8 NCHPPD.

Nurse practitioner staffing is difficult to quantify and there are few accepted guidelines for inpatient care. Hours of coverage and job responsibilities are the best indicator of need but will vary considerably across institutions.

THE MULTIDISCIPLINARY TEAM

Patients with HF benefit from a multidisciplinary approach to care. According to Coons and Fera,[4] multidisciplinary programs are required for patients at high risk for hospital admission or clinical deterioration because they facilitate the implementation of practice guidelines, attack barriers related to compliance with treatment plans, and reduce the risk of repeated hospitalization.[4] In addition, multidisciplinary teams have played an essential role in implementing evidence-based performance measures for heart failure as required by the Joint Commission on Accreditation of Healthcare Organizations (JCAHO).[9]

The Heart Failure Unit and Team

A HF unit is designed to cluster patients with heart failure and to better manage the disease process by providing efficient and timely patient-centered care and education. The heart failure unit has a designated Medical Director who is the gatekeeper for heart failure admissions. The Medical Director must maintain control of patient flow in and out of the unit and is responsible for placing complex heart failure patients appropriately.

Central to the success of the HF unit, is a strong and well functioning team. The multidisciplinary team is active 7 days a week and is instrumental in delivery of high-quality, efficient care. The members of the team include: cardiologist, NPs, pharmacist, physical therapist, registered dietician, social worker, bedside nurses, and nursing care coordinator. Figure 18.6 depicts the relationships of the team members and defines the responsibilities of individual team members.

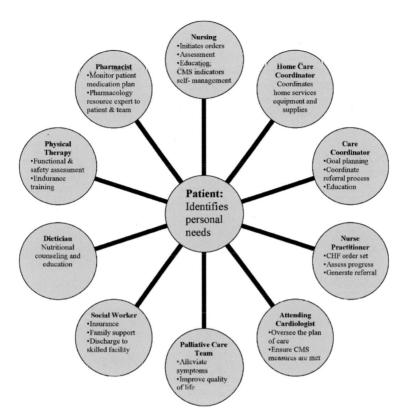

FIGURE 18.6. Roles of interdisciplinary heart failure team.

The focus of the team is to ensure that:

- JCAHO evidenced-based CMS measures are met.
- Standardized educational needs are implemented.
- The treatment plan is appropriate based on individualized needs of the patient.
- Referrals are initiated.
- A safe discharge plan is provided.
- Follow-up appointments are established prior to discharge.

The multidisciplinary team is large and each member contributes to the overall plan for the patient. The greatest challenge to the team is maintaining communication throughout hospitalization. The "huddle" is referenced earlier in this chapter as an effective means to augment communication about patient care. It serves another important function by providing a means for continuous quality improvement. The team shares what works well and what does not work well. Improvements in patient care processes (such as hand-offs, med reconciliation, and rapid response) can be discussed and implemented using a rapid cycle improvement methodology. The team becomes fully responsible for the care being provided and the outcomes of that care.

OUTCOMES

Cohorting complex heart failure patients on one unit with a team of professionals who specialize in heart failure management can make a significant impact on patient care outcomes. In our academic medical center, after the introduction of a multidisciplinary HFTT, CMS measures are consistently above the hospital average and the national average with the most recent scores showing outstanding achievement:

* 100% compliance with discharge instructions
* 100% compliance with ACE/ARB
* 100% compliance with echocardiogram
* 100% compliance with smoking cessation

Press Ganey patient satisfaction scores are consistently greater than 90% which is above the hospital mean and in line with national standards.

The HFTT care model exemplifies a true multidisciplinary team approach with clear and measurable benefits for patients, providers, and systems.

References

1. American Heart Association (2004) Heart and stroke statistics update. American Heart Association, Dallas, TX.
2. Graves E, Owings M (1998) Advance data from vital and health statistics. National Hospital Discharge Survey. DHSS publication No. PHS 98-1250: 1–12. Public Health Service, Hyattsville, MD.
3. Regan, R (2008) Heart failure. In: Buttaro T, Trybulski J, Baily P, Sandberg-Cook J (eds) Primary care: a collaborative practice, 3rd edn. Mosby, St. Louis, MO.
4. Coons J, Fera T (2007) Practice Report; Multidisciplinary team for enhancing care for patients with acute myocardial infarction or heart failure. American Journal of Health-System Pharmacy 64:1274–1277.
5. Senni M, Rodeheffer R, Tribouilloy C (1999) Use of echocardiography in the management of congestive heart failure in the community. Journal of the American College of Cardiology 33:164–170.

6. Berkowitz R, Blank L, Powell, S (2005) Strategies to reduce hospitalizations in the management of heart failure. Lippincott's Case Management, Supplement to Volume 10 10(6S):S1–S15.
7. Hunt S, Baker D, Chin, M (2001) ACC/AHA guidelines for the evaluation and management of chronic heart failure in the adult: A report to the American College of Cardiology/American Heart Association task force on practice guidelines. American College of Cardiology. http://www.acc.org/clinical/guidelines/failure/hf_index.htm.
8. Kimmelstiel C, DeNofrio D, Konstam M (2005) Heart failure. In: Wachter R, Goldman, L, Hollander H (eds) Hospital medicine, 2nd edn. Lippincott, Williams & Wilkins, Philadelphia, PA.
9. Aplesh A, Owen M (2006) Productive interdisciplinary team relationships. Lippincott's Case Management 11(3):106–164.

Chapter 19
Physical Activity in Heart Failure

Vicki Malzewski and Laurie Kopin

INTRODUCTION

Symptoms of fatigue and dyspnea with minimal exertion are both common symptoms that prompt patients to seek medical care. Oftentimes, these patients are diagnosed with varying degrees of congestive heart failure (HF) depending on the advancement of the disease process. In the past, patients diagnosed with congestive HF were excluded from formal exercise programs and discouraged from participating in any type of physical activity because of concerns about detrimental effects on an already weakened heart.[1,2] It was thought that the disease progression coupled with severe deconditioning and reduced skeletal muscle mass[3,4] only serve to exacerbate HF symptoms. In addition to high morbidity and mortality rates, it is not uncommon for this patient population to have a very low functional capacity, a decreased perceived quality of life (QOL), and some degree of anxiety and/or depression.[5,6] We now know that among the numerous physiological and psychological benefits HF patients receive from physical activity, recent studies have also shown a decrease in hospital admissions[3] and adverse cardiac events,[7] as well as decreased morbidity and mortality[8,9] following a structured exercise training program. It was not until recently that structured exercise became one of the cornerstones of beneficial treatment modalities used to treat HF patients. Recent initiatives such as the National Institutes of Health (NIH) HF-Action[1] trial are seeking to scientifically support the overwhelming, holistic benefits that exercise has on these patients.

J.D. Bisognano et al. (eds.), *Manual of Heart Failure Management*,
DOI: 10.1007/978-1-84882-185-9_19, © Springer-Verlag London Limited 2009

FACTORS AFFECTING EXERCISE INTOLERANCE

HF is characterized by a reduced exercise tolerance and early fatigability. The ability to perform aerobic activity depends on both an increase in cardiac output (CO) to working muscles and the capability of these muscles to utilize the oxygen delivered by the blood. Therefore, maximal oxygen consumption (VO_2max) = CO × arteriovenous oxygen (AVO_2) difference. A reduced aerobic capacity is largely the result of inadequate blood supply to active muscles secondary to reduced CO. A lower maximum heart rate achieved at a lower workload coupled with only minimal increases in stroke volume results in an inability to increase CO sufficiently. In fact, patients with HF may only achieve <50% of the peak CO achieved by a healthy person at maximal exercise.[10]

In addition to cardiovascular abnormalities affecting exercise intolerance, there are several peripheral factors, which must also be considered. Patients with chronic HF have a reduction in the release of nitric oxide, normally stimulated by exercise in healthy individuals, which is imperative as a mediator for peripheral vasodilatation and thus, for tissue perfusion. Also, peripheral vascular resistance fails to decrease with exercise in HF patients leading to preferential blood flow to nonexercising tissues and hypoperfusion of exercising muscle.[10,11] It is this combination of cardiovascular and peripheral impairments that ultimately leads to a reduced AVO_2 difference, a lower peak VO_2, and severely reduced exercise capacity.

BENEFITS OF EXERCISE TRAINING IN HEART FAILURE PATIENTS

As the paradigm has shifted from exercise restriction to exercise encouragement in this patient population, many studies have shown the overwhelming benefits of structured exercise programs. Increased exercise duration and VO_2max have been shown following varying lengths of physical rehabilitation.[3,7,10] Several studies have demonstrated an increase, albeit modest, in left ventricular ejection fraction as well as an antiremodeling effect.[4,11,12] An inverse relationship exists between increasing physical fitness level and heart rate response. As physical fitness increases, resting and peak exercise heart rate decrease[3] as well as decreased ventilation and perceived dyspnea at a given workload.[10] Exercise training has been shown to increase the number of muscle mitochondria, the organelle responsible for energy production, thus delaying the switch to anaerobic metabolism.[10] As patients increase activity, there is a decrease in their symptoms, as well as a decrease in their anxiety level regarding exercise.[5] With strength training comes an increase in muscle mass and contractile strength,[3,12] which often leads to an increased ability to perform the activities of daily life (ADL) with less difficulty and fatigue[2] and an increase in the patient's QOL. Perhaps the most notable benefit of exercise training in these patients is the decrease in the number of hospitalizations and increased survival rates. Dracup et al. examined the effects of a home-based exercise program on clinical outcomes. They found patients in the control group required nearly twice as many hospitalizations over the one year follow-up period as the exercise group.[13] Belardinelli et al. demonstrated reduced rates of hospitalizations and cardiac mortality in patients randomized to 14 months of aerobic training as compared to the control group.[14] It is widely recognized that confirmation is required from a large clinical trial, which is statistically powered to examine the effects of exercise training on morbidity and mortality in these patients. The ongoing landmark clinical trial sponsored by the NIH, the HF-ACTION trial (Heart Failure and A Controlled Trial Investigating Outcomes of Exercise Training) seeks to do just that. With results due out in 2008, it is the largest of its kind, enrolling 3,000 patients with NYHA classes II to IV heart failure symptoms. The objective of this trial is to establish whether exercise training reduces all-cause mortality or all-cause hospitalizations in this group of patients.[1] The results of this study are eagerly awaited, and will hopefully add much-needed data in this area.

RISKS OF EXERCISE TRAINING IN HEART FAILURE PATIENTS

As with all patient populations, there are potential risks associated with exercise training. In patients with HF, there are greater rates of morbidity and mortality when compared with healthy individuals. Therefore, current guidelines dictate patients with HF be considered at the highest level of risk. The most common exercise-related events in such patients include atrial and ventricular arrhythmias, worsening heart failure symptoms, and post exercise hypotension. Myocardial infarction (MI) is another risk associated with involvement in exercise training, as is sudden cardiac death, albeit much less likely. It is important to note the adjusted relative risk of MI has been found to be greater in persons who do not exercise regularly when compared with those who regularly participate in physical activity.[10] A thoughtful and cautious approach to the initiation of a structured exercise program should be used with HF patients. The exercise program should be individualized with a thorough health history and physical assessment performed prior to the commencement of exercise. The patient's functional

TABLE 19.1. Absolute and relative contraindications to exercise in patients with stable HF

Absolute contraindications	Relative contraindications
Acute myocardial infarction (<2 days)	Significant weight gain over prior 1–3 days
High-risk unstable angina	Decrease in systolic BP with exercise
Decompensated heart failure	NYHA functional class IV
Uncontrolled cardiac arrhythmias, new a-fib	Complex ventricular arrhythmia at rest
Acute myocarditis or pericarditis	Supine resting HR ^{3} 100 bpm
Severe aortic stenosis	Preexisting comorbidities
Significant ischemia at low workloads	Outflow tract obstruction (HOCM)
Uncontrolled hypertension	Significant valvular regurgitation
Acute systemic illness (pulmonary embolism, aortic dissection)	Physical impairment with inability to exercise safely

capacity with consideration of the HF class should ideally be used when formulating the exercise prescription. It goes without saying, it is imperative the prescribed supervised exercise program have a strong educational component that will not only enhance the safety and quality of exercise, but also patient compliance. A thorough and individualized approach will ultimately enhance the overall benefit to the patient (Table 19.1).

BARRIERS TO COMPLIANCE WITH PRESCRIBED EXERCISE PROGRAMS

Compliance is crucial to obtain maximal benefits from any exercise program. It is estimated that up to one third of patients who participate in exercise studies are found to be noncompliant with the exercise protocol.[15] HF patients tend to have preexisting comorbidities, which may make exercising difficult. These may include peripheral arterial disease, neuromuscular disorders, arthritis, ischemic heart disease, or diabetes.[15] Some elderly patients may feel they are too old to benefit from an exercise program, even though debilitated older patients stand to have the greatest gains in their functional status and QOL from exercise training.[3] As the duration of HF symptoms increase, patients tend to have more time to consider their prognosis and question whether an exercise program holds promise for them. When an activity, whether it be smoking cessation, dietary modifications or exercise is seen as being of little benefit, it is less likely to be performed, according to the Champion's Health Belief Model.[15] Anxiety also plays a key role in noncompliance with exercise programs. HF patients are often concerned and anxious about their ability to take part in physical activities. Anxiety can cause an increase in heart rate and stress levels, which leads to a spiraling process of growing apprehension. Depression may also limit physical activity whether or not the individual's health is a limiting factor.[6] Supervision and education are crucial to success in these patients. Financial constraints must also be considered when discussing barriers to compliance. Exercise training is not currently cost reimbursed by the Centers for Medicare and Medicaid for cardiac rehabilitation services for HF patients in the absence of an ischemic event. This can leave a large financial burden for the patient who wants to benefit from supervised exercise training without insurance to defray the cost.[4] Logistical factors such as a lack of transportation, climate concerns, time conflicts, and lack of access to equipment or facilities are also sometimes a problem. A greater number of home or community-based programs, as opposed to hospital-based programs, may help overcome these obstacles, be more cost-effective, and allow for greater flexibility for the patient.[3]

ASSESSMENT OF EXERCISE CAPACITY

Cardiopulmonary exercise testing (CPET) is widely used in the evaluation of patients with systolic HF because it is probably the single most important predictor of prognosis in HF patients as it assesses VO_2max while exercising. HF patients with a VO_2max <13 ml kg^{-1} min^{-1} had a yearly mortality of 36% when compared with patients with a VO_2max of >13 ml kg^{-1} min^{-1} who had a 15% mortality.[16] During exercise, the cardiovascular system performs gas exchange, delivering oxygen to working muscles and extracting carbon dioxide and other metabolites. CPET measures fractions of oxygen and carbon dioxide in expired gas during exercise by using a mask or mouthpiece at the patient's mouth. Samples of expired air are collected every 15 s with real-time data expressed in graph or tabular form. Many laboratories use ramping protocols on either the treadmill or bicycle. This allows for the workload to increase in a constant or continuous fashion to accommodate a wide range of patient capabilities while still keeping the test within the desired time frame of 8–12 min.[17] For example, a 10 W ramping bicycle protocol would gradually increase resistance by 10 W over each minute of exercise. Naughton or Balke-Ware treadmill protocols can also be utilized, as they involve only minor increases in elevation at a fixed speed. Ideally, an exercise prescription should be formulated based on information gained from a CPET, with routine follow-up CPET to track progress and adjust the exercise

TABLE 19.2. Borg rating of perceived exertion

6 No exertion at all
7 Extremely light
8
9 Very light
10
11 Light
12
13 Somewhat hard
14
15 Hard
16
17 Very hard
18
19 Extremely hard
20 Maximal exertion

prescription accordingly. If metabolic stress testing is not possible, submaximal tests such as the 6-min walk test (6MWT) can be used to determine appropriate exercise intensity. The 6MWT is a self-paced test where the patient is encouraged to walk as far as possible within the allotted 6-min time frame. The distance covered is used to approximate functional capacity.

The Borg scale of Rating of Perceived Exertion (RPE) is another way to measure intensities both for formulating an exercise prescription, and for patient self-monitoring during exercise sessions (Table 19.2). This is especially useful in patients who do not have a normal heart rate response to exercise due to medications or other factors. The patient simply correlates how hard they feel when they are working with the corresponding number on the scale.

RECOMMENDATIONS FOR EXERCISE TRAINING IN HEART FAILURE

Before embarking on an exercise training program, Class II and III HF patients should be on stable and optimal medical therapy for at least a month, and have their medical history and current state of health scrutinized.[2,16] The list of absolute and relative contraindications should be reviewed by the clinician and with the patient to ensure safety. A brief supervised period should take place, when possible, to facilitate patient education, monitor vital signs during activity, track progress, and provide social support from staff and fellow patients. This period also serves to increase the patient's confidence in his or her ability to exercise safely and effectively.[10]

Ideally, the patient will continue to attend a supervised cardiac rehabilitation program when possible, or can transition to a home program. The patient should have regular follow-up visits with their healthcare provider to monitor progress, have questions answered, and have modifications made to the exercise prescription to accommodate increases in exercise tolerance and muscle strength. A strong emphasis should be placed on individualization for each patient. There is no blanket exercise prescription that works for all patients with HF.[9] An exercise program should meet the individual needs and goals of the patient while utilizing information gained from an exercise stress test as an objective assessment of functional capacity. The most frequent exercise intensity range is 60–80% of VO_2max.[10,16] For patients who are severely debilitated, a lower intensity and more frequent periods of rest may be required initially until adequate conditioning allows for increased workloads for longer periods of time. All exercise sessions should start with a warm-up period of 10–15 min of light activity and stretching, and end with a brief cool-down. A variety of exercise modalities utilizing large muscle groups can be employed, with biking and walking being the most common. Training on various pieces of equipment can be performed as continuous, interval, or a combination of both. In addition to aerobic conditioning, moderate resistance training should be encouraged to increase skeletal muscle mass and strength and ultimately make day-to-day tasks less fatiguing.[12] Small free weights, weighing 1–2 lbs, or elastic bands are easy for patients to use at home, and are inexpensive to acquire. The exercise program should take into account the patient's access to programs or facilities, time constraints, physical abilities with regard to different modalities, and their activities of choice to optimize the likelihood of compliance. It is important to note swimming is not recommended in this patient population due to an increased pulmonary capillary wedge pressure and acute volume loading on the left ventricle caused by hydrostatic pressure when immersed in water[2] (Table 19.3).

A cardiac rehabilitation setting is ideal venue for initiating HF patients into an exercise program because of the complexity and high number of variables to consider along with the crucial need for individualization and close follow-up by a multidisciplinary team of healthcare professionals. If attendance at a formal rehabilitation setting is not possible, a home-based program should be encouraged. This should include specific, uninterrupted exercise for at least 20–30 min 4–5 days per week. Special care should be taken to provide information to these patients on self-monitoring, optimizing safety, and signs and symptoms that should prompt a

TABLE 19.3. Exercise prescription guidelines

	Aerobic-continuous	Aerobic-interval	Resistance training
Frequency: sessions/wk	2–6	2–6	2–3
Intensity % peak VO_2	Initially 50–60% increase to 60–80%	Initially 50–60% increase to 60–90%	N/A
Intensity % peak HR	55–75%	55–85%	70–75% 1 repetition max
Repetitions per session	1	15–30	6–10 per set-build up to 3 sets
Minutes per session	Initially 10–20 increase to 20–30	30–60 s	15–30

TABLE 19.4. Patient education

General Information
- Explanation of heart failure
- Role of family as support

Benefits of Exercise Training
- Overall health
- Quality of Life

Self-Monitoring
- Daily weight measurement
- Blood pressure/HR monitoring
- Common symptoms

Safety
- Never exercise alone
- When to call the Doctor
- When not to exercise

Exercise Guidelines
- Initiation with gradual progression
- Symptom-limiting
- Taking rest days when needed
- Maintaining active lifestyle for life

call to their health care provider. Patients should feel confident in their ability to exercise safely, and understand that adhering to their exercise prescription is vitally important to their overall health and safety (Table 19.4).

CONCLUSION

Until recently, regular physical activity was, for the most part, discouraged in the HF population. However, an increasing number of clinical trials have demonstrated the many benefits exercise provides in these patients. In addition to physiologic changes such as decreased HF symptoms, decreased anxiety, increase in muscle mass, and increased ability to perform ADLs, studies have shown cost benefits in the form of reduced hospitalizations and decreased mortality among regularly active HF patients. Initiating patients into a formal exercise program requires a multidisciplinary team approach to aid in patient education and encourage consistency. Patients should clearly understand the benefits such activity will provide, as well as the importance of sustaining an active lifestyle indefinitely.

Ideally, patients should begin exercising in a monitored environment, such as a cardiac rehabilitation facility, with progression to a home program. Exercise prescriptions should be highly individualized and preferentially based on information gained from a CPET. Provisions should be made to provide close follow-up with adaptations to the regimen as needed. When appropriate, a comprehensive exercise program should include both aerobic exercise and light strength training. Patients should be counseled on strategies to maximize safety to decrease anxiety about exercise and increase patient confidence when exercising independently.

Patient education and understanding regarding exercise is an important key to success in this patient population. This highlights the clinician's role in creating an exercise prescription that is highly individualized, taking into consideration any patient limitations, and provides ongoing support and encouragement to increase the likelihood of lifetime compliance.

References

1. Whellan D, O'Conner C, Lee K et al. (2007) Heart Failure and A Controlled Trial Investigating Outcomes of Exercise TraiNing (HF-ACTION): Design and rationale. American Heart Journal 153:201–211.
2. Wise F (2007) Exercise based cardiac rehabilitation in chronic heart failure. Australian Family Physician 36:1019–1024.
3. Fleg J (2007) Exercise therapy for elderly heart failure patients. Clinics in Geriatric Medicine 23:221–234.
4. Rubin S (2007) Exercise training in heart failure. Journal of the American College of Cardiology 49:2337–2340.
5. Kulcu D, Kurtais Y, Tur B et al. (2007) The effect of cardiac rehabilitation on quality of life, anxiety and depression in patients with congestive heart failure. A randomized controlled trial, short term results. Europa Medicophysica 43:489–497.

6. McMahon K, Lip Y (2002) Psychological factors in heart failure. Archives of Internal Medicine 162:509–516.

7. Mueller L, Myers J, Kottman W et al. (2007) Exercise capacity, physical activity patterns and outcomes six years after cardiac rehabilitation in patients with heart failure. Clinical Rehabilitation 21:923–931.

8. Haykowsky M, Yuanyuan L, Pechter D et al. (2007) A meta-analysis of the effect of exercise training on left ventricular remodeling in heart failure patients. Journal of the American College of Cardiology 49:2329–2336.

9. Ko J, McKelvie R (2005) The role of exercise training for patients with heart failure. Europa Medicophysica 41:35–47.

10. Pina I, Apstein C, Balady G et al. (2003) Exercise and heart failure: A Statement From the American Heart Association Committee on Exercise, Rehabilitation and Prevention. Circulation 107:1210–1225.

11. Keteyian S (2006) Exercise rehabilitation in chronic heart failure. Coronary Artery Disease 17:233–237.

12. Feiereisen P, Delagardelle C, Vaillant M et al. (2007) Is strength training the more efficient training modality in chronic heart failure? Medicine and Science in Sports and Exercise 39:1910–1917.

13. Dracup K, Evangelista L, Hamilton M et al. (2007) Effects of a home-based exercise program on clinical outcomes in heart failure. American Heart Journal 154:877–883.

14. Belardinelli R, Georgiou D, Cianci G et al. (1999) Randomized, controlled trial of long-term moderate exercise training in chronic heart failure: effects on functional capacity, quality of life, and clinical outcome. Circulation 99:1173–1182.

15. Covera-Tindel T, Doering L, Gomez T et al. (2004) Predictors of Noncompliance in Heart Failure. Journal of Cardiovascular Nursing 19:269–277.

16. Smart N, Fang Z, Marwick T (2003) A practical guide to exercise training for heart failure patients. Journal of Cardiac Failure 9:49–58.

17. Milani R, Lavie C, Mehra M et al. (2006) Understanding the basics of cardiopulmonary exercise testing. Mayo Clinic Proceedings 81:1603–1611.

Index